Strength Training for Seniors Over 60

Simple Home Workouts to Restore Balance, Improve Mobility and Rebuild Muscle so you can perform daily activities with ease

Gerald B. Coleman RN, JD

Contents

Introduction

We were told growing up that exercise is good for our health. However, the older you get, the more critical it is to stay physically active because it protects you from the health issues associated with aging or reduces their severity.

I imagine you still want to feel good, perform the simple daily tasks you've been doing over the years, run around with your grandchildren, and spend more time with your loved ones.

You need strength to do all these.

The good news is that you can still have this active and healthy lifestyle by adopting strength training.

Our strength and muscle mass diminish as we age, and this condition is referred to as sarcopenia. Studies show that our muscle mass declines by about 3% to 8% every ten years from when we turn 30 and worsens when we reach 60.

When our muscle mass and strength decrease, we are vulnerable to falls and injury, and we start relying on those around us to help us with daily tasks like walking and carrying groceries, among others.

These changes also put us at risk for osteoporosis, diabetes, cardiovascular disease, and high blood pressure.

Yes, these changes come with age. However, lack of exercise makes them worse.

This is where strength training comes in.

While strength training cannot stop the aging process, it can slow it down and thus delay or reduce some of its effects on the body.

In fact, studies show that strength training is among the top ways to combat the weakness associated with aging.

The role of strength training is to help your body form and maintain muscles, therefore reversing the negative health issues we've discussed above.

Strength training involves using some resistance, like weights, dumbbells, or resistance bands. That's how you improve your strength and stability and regain or maintain your independence. Therefore, activities like walking or cycling fall outside this category.

Resistance training exercises strengthen your upper body (chest, shoulders, back) and lower body (thighs, backside, and lower leg). We'll talk about this more in the book.

Engaging in strength training also improves your mood and emotional and mental well-being. You need to do these exercises regularly to experience the benefits.

You may have questions about where to start. I have created this book, Strength Training for Seniors: Restore Balance, Improve Mobility, and Rebuild Muscle, to help you learn how to do strength training safely and effectively to build strength/muscle, improve your health, and live a healthy lifestyle.

If you are wondering whether this book is for you, ask yourself whether you fall into any of these categories:

You want to become physically fit to protect yourself from old age-related illness and live a healthy life.

You want to be active so you can have the strength to interact with your family and friends.

You've tried working out but have yet to experience visible results.

You want to engage in strength training exercises but fear you may not execute them properly.

You want to exercise, but the gym isn't your favorite place, so you're looking for simple yet effective at-home workouts.

You've encountered bits of information on strength training scattered over the internet, but you prefer a one-stop reading resource with all the details you need.

You are in the right place if you answered yes to any of these questions.

And don't worry if you have long-term illnesses like arthritis, high blood pressure, or diabetes. You can still safely practice strength training and reap the mentioned benefits, just like everyone else. Just make sure you doctor before beginning any exercise program.

By reading this book, you'll learn why you need to exercise, the numerous health benefits of incorporating exercise into your life, how often you need to exercise, simple strength training workouts you can do at home, and safety tips to help you prevent injuries while working out.

It doesn't matter if you haven't been active in the previous years or have not worked out regularly. By reading this book, you are choosing to live a healthier lifestyle, and anyone can do that regardless of their age, gender, or how active they have been previously.

Congratulations on starting the journey to a stronger, healthier, more vibrant, and independent YOU.

Let's dive in!

Chapter 1
The Body As We Age

It's like looking straight at a stranger.

That's what Hayley felt as she looked at herself intently in the mirror. Wasn't it just yesterday when she looked and felt like a million bucks?

Just like her ancestors before her, Hayley was blessed with the kind of good looks that make men stand up and take notice. She had thick and glossy dark hair that was the envy of many.

Her skin was as smooth as silk; men and women envied her young-looking skin.

She had the kind of body you only see on magazine covers. She brings style to a whole new level.

Hayley exuded charm and grace. But most of all, she was strong and fit.

But as the years went by, she changed.

She started to notice fine lines growing on her face. Then, her hairline began to recede, and the shiny black color started to fade.

She had to wear reading glasses. Her 20-20 vision has left the building.

Then, she noticed that she got weaker and weaker. Even the most minor task can wear her out in an instant.

What happened to her?

The answer is obvious - AGING caught up with her.

Changes In the Body With Aging

Let's face it. Aging is a part of life. Whether we like it or not, we will go through that phase.

That phase will involve changes in our bodies. Aging causes the body to alter because both individual cells and entire organs change. The function and appearance of cells are altered due to these adjustments.

For people to be able to handle these changes, it is best to be knowledgeable about them. It is vital to have a clear understanding of what one goes through.

So, let's look at how aging affects our bodies.

Aging Cells

Cells become less efficient as they get older. To make way for new cells, old cells must die. This cycle is all a part of the grand design.

Cells' genes perform a process that, when activated, causes the cell to die. Apoptosis, a type of cell suicide, is this type of planned demise.

Cells can only divide a finite number of times, another reason they expire. Genes pre-program this limit, and a cell that cannot divide eventually dies.

Aging organs

A component known as a telomere is responsible for the mechanism that restricts cell division. Telomeres transfer the genetic material to prepare the cell for cell division. The telomeres get slightly shorter each time a cell divides, and the telomeres eventually get so short that the cell can't divide. Senescence refers to the process in which a cell ceases to divide.

Cells get damaged. Here are some of the reasons behind it:

* Exposure to harmful substances like too much sunlight, chemotherapy drugs, and radiation.

* Free radicals

Oxygen-containing molecules with an unbalanced number of electrons are known as free radicals, and they can easily interact with other molecules because of their unequal quantity. Free radicals can produce lengthy chemical chains in your body because they interact quickly with other molecules.

As the body ages, the number of cells in the ovaries, testes, kidneys, and liver drops noticeably. A low cell count prevents an organ from functioning correctly. As a result, most organs evolve and can be less efficient.

Not every organ, though, has a significant cell loss. One illustration is the brain. Healthy seniors do not have significant brain cell loss. Significant losses primarily affect stroke survivors or those with neurodegenerative diseases like Parkinson's or Alzheimer's that cause substantial degeneration in nerve cells.

Frequently, the musculoskeletal system exhibits the first aging symptoms. Early in mid-life, the eyes and ears start to change.

In general, internal processes get worse as we age. Before age 30, most physical processes peak, and after that, they diminish gradually but continuously.

Despite this loss, most functions remain sufficient because most organs begin life with significantly more functional ability than the body requires. This ability is referred to as functional reserve.

Even if most functions continue to be acceptable, age-related function decreases, making older persons less able to deal with various stimuli, such as demanding physical exercise, abrupt temperature changes, and disorders. This reduction indicates that elderly individuals are more susceptible to adverse pharmacological effects.

Under stress, some organs are more inclined to malfunction compared to others. These include the brain, urinary organs, blood vessels, kidneys, heart, and brain.

Bones and Joints

You can expect your bones to become less dense at a certain age. Osteopenia occurs when there is moderate loss of bone density, and osteoporosis occurs when the loss is severe.

When you have osteoporosis, your bones weaken, making them more likely to break. When menopause hits, the loss of bone density among women becomes quicker, and the reason for this is less estrogen production.

What are estrogens? They are a group of hormones playing a crucial role in the reproductive and sexual development of females, and they are also called sex hormones.

A woman's ovaries are the leading creators of most estrogen hormones. The fat cells and adrenal glands are responsible for making small amounts.

Why are estrogens important? They are considered so because they prevent too much bone from breaking during the body's forming, breaking down, and re-forming routine.

One of the primary reasons bones experience less density is a lack of calcium. Calcium is a mineral essential for bone health, and it is also necessary to maintain the proper functioning of our muscular, cardiovascular, and nervous systems.

There are three bones in our body that weaken the most often:

- The femur or the end of the thigh bone

- Vertebrae or the spine bones

- Radius and Ulna or the ends of the arm bones

Let's look into the vertebrae a bit further. When there are changes at the top of your spine, they may cause your head to tip a bit forward. This head tilting results in throat compression, making it difficult to swallow and susceptible to choking.

It's common knowledge that when people get older, they get shorter. This is because the cushions of bone tissues lose fluid, making them thinner, eventually shortening the spine.

Years of movement result in the cartilage becoming thin. A joint's surface cannot slide over one another as well as before, so the joint becomes more susceptible to breaks and injuries.

Muscles and Body Fat

Osteoarthritis is one of the most common bone conditions in a person's later years. The most significant factor in this is damage to the cartilage brought upon by repeated injury or lifelong use.

Ligaments bind our joints; our muscles are attached to our bones by tendons. Ligaments and tendons lose elasticity when one gets older. Do you experience joint tightness and stiffness? Well, now you know why those occur.

Older people become less physically flexible. Their tendons and ligaments tear more quickly and heal more slowly.

Typically, muscle mass or the amount of our muscle tissue begins to decline by the time we reach 30 years old. The same goes for muscle strength.

Some of the reasons for this are:

- Physical inactivity or a sedentary lifestyle

- A decrease in hormone or testosterone growth

- Slow-contracting muscles

According to MSD Manual, about 10 to 15 percent of muscle mass is reduced due to aging. But it is good to note that that percentage can be prevented through regular activities such as exercise. But more on that later.

Eyes

As we reach middle age, the lens of our eyes becomes less flexible, and it is also less able to thicken. This situation brings about focus issues on nearby objects, which is called presbyopia. You might need bifocals or reading glasses for this.

Other eye issues that occur due to aging are the following:

- Conjunctiva thinning

- Browning/yellowing of the lens

- Decrease in tear production resulting in dry eyes.

- Decrease in the count of mucous cells.

- Arcus senilis, or a deposit of cholesterol salts and calcium

Retina diseases are likely to happen in old age. These include:

- Diabetic retinopathy

- Macular degeneration (if the person has diabetes)

- Cataracts

- Detachment of one's retina

Ears

While not a primary reason, aging is a factor in hearing loss. Hearing changes happen as one ages, and this condition is called Presbycusis.

Did you know that high-pitched noises and sounds are challenging to hear for older adults? The violin is an instrument that has a high-pitched sound. But due to Presbycusis, the music tends to sound less bright.

In Presbycusis, words and phrases become more challenging to understand. Sometimes, it appears like other people are mumbling, although, in reality, they usually speak understandably.

Most consonants, such as the letters "t," "k," "p," and "ch," are high-pitched. Older people need others to articulate their consonants clearly instead of speaking louder, which is a common misconception when talking to older people.

Mouth and Nose

As one gets older, the quality of taste and smell are also affected. These senses diminish, making it harder for people to appreciate food.

It would help if you had a strong sense of taste and smell to enjoy a range of flavors from your foods. So, when they diminish, it can be frustrating not to be able to fully identify even the most basic tastes, such as sweet, bitter, salty, and sour. If you must know, your sense of smell is crucial to determine more complex and subtle flavors. An example of this is raspberry.

When one reaches their older years, taste buds decrease in sensitivity, especially with sweets and salty foods. Also, the ability to smell is affected, and that's because the lining of your nose becomes drier and thinner as the nerve endings begin to deteriorate.

Your mouth frequently feels dry because you produce less saliva. A dry mouth further exacerbates the issues with taste.

Here are other noticeable signs:

- The gums recede a bit.

- Tooth enamel wears away.

- Teeth are more prone to cavities and decay.

- The nose enlarges and lengthens with the tip drooping.

- Thick hairs appear on the nose.

Skin

The skin ultimately becomes thinner, drier, less elastic, and wrinkled. These situations occur because collagen and elastin become less flexible and are chemically changed.

Collagen is a group of proteins found in the skin's connective tissue. According to skincraft. com, almost 30% of a person's body protein is collagen.

Conversely, elastin is a fibroblast protein that forms a chain of elastic fibers. These fibers ensure the skin's firmness and elasticity.

Wrinkles develop when the skin's fat layer thins. This layer's role is to be a cushion to protect the skin—loose and saggy skin results when the fat in the deeper parts of your skin diminishes. There are also more-pronounced crevices and lines.

All five primary sensations (touch, pain, itch, warmth, and cold) can be produced by sensory nerve endings in the skin. When these nerve endings decrease, individuals injure themselves easily.

Blood flow in the inner layers of the skin declines, along with the number of sweat glands and blood vessels. Due to this, the body has a more challenging time transferring heat from inside through its blood vessels to its surface.

Because the body fails to yield heat, it cannot chill itself as effectively. This situation leads to a higher risk of heat-related diseases, including heatstroke. Furthermore, the skin tends to recover more slowly when the blood supply is reduced.

The number of melanocytes or pigment-producing cells also decreases with age. The skin has less protection against ultraviolet (UV) radiation. Age spots develop on one's skin when exposed to sunlight because the skin is less capable of removing waste products.

The skin becomes less able to form Vitamin D from sunlight. Therefore, a person's risk of developing vitamin D deficiency increases.

Brain and the Nervous System

The number of nerve cells in our brain declines when aging hits, and some levels of the chemical substances, which are the means of sending messages to the brain, decrease. That's because nerve cells lose some receptors needed to transmit messages.

Decreased blood flow to the brain is a chronic change that transpires as a person ages. Such a situation does not usually come with symptoms. But frequent occurrences may result in gradual brain tissue deterioration that will affect a person's cognitive functions, including the ability to learn new information, short-term memory, the ability to recall words, and vocabulary use.

Heart and Blood Vessels

Have you noticed your heart not beating as fast during physical exertion? Aging does that. It can cause changes in your heart and blood vessels.

It's during this time when the heart and blood vessels become stiffer. Unlike when we were younger, our arteries cannot expand as they used to when blood is pumped through, resulting in the heart filling with blood slowly.

The outcome? High blood pressure.

Changes in the heart and blood vessels increase one's risk of heart disease. A primary factor in heart disease is the buildup of fatty deposits in the arteries walls of arteries for an extended period.

Anyone can have a heart attack, but age is a significant factor. Older individuals have a higher risk.

This risk is not only from having a heart attack. It also applies to coronary heart disease, stroke, and heart failure. All this can lead to disability, affecting your quality of life.

Lungs and Breathing Muscles

The diaphragm is a significant body muscle found just below the lungs. It's the muscle for respiration.

The diaphragm is a massive muscle shaped like a dome. It contracts continuously and rhythmically; most of the time, it does so involuntarily. When inhaling, it contracts and flattens, enlarging the chest cavity.

Apart from the diaphragm, the muscles between the ribs are used for breathing, and both tend to weaken during aging.

The number of alveoli or air sacs and capillaries in the lungs declines. This situation prevents people from absorbing oxygen as they breathe in the air. The lungs lose some elasticity, making it hard to breathe in high altitudes and making exercising a bit challenging.

The ability to fight infection is lessened due to the cells' inability to sweep debris with microorganisms out of the airways. Surprisingly, coughing clears out the lungs. But this also weakens.

Digestive System

The tube connecting the mouth to the stomach is the esophagus. This tube slows down its function when aging hits, creating a problem with swallowing food and liquids.

Since the esophagus muscles are less forceful when contracting, the stomach empties the food slowly. The stomach's elasticity prevents it from holding much food.

Some older people experience issues with their digestive tracts. One of those problems is the production of lactase.

Lactase is a body enzyme necessary for the body to digest milk. But aging sometimes causes the digestive tract to produce less lactase, resulting in lactose intolerance.

Those who are lactose intolerant cannot fully digest the sugar in milk or other milk products. If they consume these products, they get diarrhea, and they also experience bloating and gas. While these symptoms are typically harmless, they can be pretty uncomfortable.

You may experience slowness of movement of contents within the large intestine. Also, there's a slight decrease in rectum contractions when it is filled with stool. Constipation is a frequent complaint when this occurs.

There also comes a problem with the liver. It becomes smaller as there is a decrease in cell number.

Blood flow tends to be less, and liver enzymes function less efficiently. With the latter, we can experience difficulty eliminating drugs and other substances from our bodies. Therefore, any side effects of these drugs linger.

Kidneys and the Urinary Tract

Because the number of cells declines, our kidneys become smaller, and there is lesser blood flow. According to the MSD Manual, around the age of 30, people's kidneys filter blood less efficiently. If this happens, one can expect that the organ will be unable to remove waste as well.

Dehydration is a frequent occurrence. The kidneys may excrete a lot of water but little salt, which often leads to dehydration.

Have you noticed that you urinate more often? That's because the changes in your urinary tract, such as an overactive bladder, prevent you from controlling urination.

Here are other changes:

- Weakened bladder muscles

- Urinary Leakage or incontinence

- Shortened urethra (women)

- Enlarged prostate (men)

Reproductive Organs

When it comes to the hormonal effects of aging, they are more evident in females than males. Remarkably, the effects are connected to menopause.

In menopause, there is a decrease in hormone levels, causing the uterus and ovaries to shrink. Vaginal tissues become thinner, less elastic, and drier. There are cases when these effects proceed to the following:

- Bleeding
- Itching
- Urinary urgency
- Pain during sex

Women's breasts lose firmness and become more fibrous. These changes prevent the easy discovery of breast lumps.

Endocrine System

Organs called glands make up our endocrine system. These glands create and release different hormones that aim at various body areas.

Aging results in a decrease in growth hormone levels, affecting muscle mass.

Aldosterone levels decline so that dehydration can occur. This hormone tells the body to retain water and salt.

Insulin is less effective; therefore, people cannot control their blood sugar levels.

Insulin allows sugar to move from our blood into cells. In these cells, sugar converts into energy.

The changes in the endocrine system increase the risk of health issues. An example of this is Type 2 Diabetes.

Blood Production

The bone marrow is responsible for producing blood cells. But as we get older, there's a decline in the amount of active bone marrow.

This situation poses a problem when a person needs extra blood cells. If you have anemia, bleeding, or infection, producing blood cells to cater to your body's needs is imperative.

Immune System

The cells in the immune system start to act more slowly, affecting their function in identifying and destroying bacteria and cancer cells and infecting microbes and other foreign substances.

This slowdown explains the following:

- Older people are prone to getting cancer.

- Vaccines sometimes are less effective on older individuals.

- Pneumonia, flu, and other infections are more prevalent among older people.

What's happening to me?

That's what Hayley asked herself as she changed due to aging. You may be asking this question yourself.

But one of the best things you can do to slow and, in some cases, reverse some of these changes is to exercise.

Exercise is not just for the young. Regardless of age, you will find many benefits to it.

Chapter 2
The Many Benefits of Exercise

It was weird.

Every time the Christmas season rolled around, Hayley felt depressed and anxious. Weren't you supposed to be jolly and cheerful this time of the year?

Her kids and grandkids will fly in to spend time with her. There are parties to attend here and there. But no matter how hard she tries, Hayley cannot get into the holiday spirit.

Ever since she turned 60, she grew restless and sulky. She was looking forward to drinking her woes away and eating fast food! She almost forgets her plight when she imagines the plate of fries and the gigantic burger served before her.

Almost.

What was bothering her?

Does she miss working?

Does she find the silence in her house, where she now lives alone, deafening?

Or is it because of the countless times she had to go to the ER or doctor checkups because of some illness or another?

Probably the last one.

All she does is worry about what's to come next. It never crossed her mind to do something about it.

Thankfully, she ran across a high school friend at the mall, Penelope. It seemed like an ordinary run-in - catching up and the like. However, it turned out to be a life-altering experience.

Her classmate was just like her - retired, widowed, and with children all grown and living far away.

The difference between them is that Penelope stays active.

She volunteers at the shelter, is active at Church, and, most importantly, is fit and healthy.

Looking at them side by side, one wouldn't be able to guess that Hayley and Penelope are both in their 60s. The latter looks so much younger - and happier!

Penelope mentioned that she decided to do strength training workouts a few years back. And she has not stopped since! She told Hayley she could do the same.

Hayley burst out laughing. "Aren't we too old for that?!" She asked incredulously.

Penelope smiled knowingly. "That's what I thought, too. But it turns out it was the best decision I made. And it would be yours also, Hayley."

Hayley decided to make a change. She did a home strength training challenge. Exercise now became a part of her routine.

The effects were gradual but effective. Not only did Hayley's depression disappear, her physical health improved-- No more ER visits or alarming lab results.

Hayley stopped her unhealthy food habits and turned her back on fast food to ramp up her new active lifestyle. She began cooking healthy meals and packing nutritious snacks, such as sliced rotisserie chicken and fresh fruits and vegetables.

Hayley gained a new perspective on life.

When she saw Penelope again, and Penelope asked her about her experience, this is what she said:

"It was an incredible blessing. While my body is not perfect, I am content with it. I didn't realize until now what exercise can do for my soul. Exercise is not just the physical stuff. It affects your mental, emotional, and spiritual well-being. It encompasses everything."

Benefits of Exercise After 60

Exercise is an activity for everyone, regardless of age. It's all-encompassing.

Here are the most notable benefits:

1 Prevents chronic illnesses.
Exercise gives off a protective curtain to keep chronic illnesses at bay. For instance, aerobic exercise raises your heart rate, improving your heart health and protecting you from cardiovascular diseases. If you already have a chronic illness, such as diabetes, physical activities will minimize the symptoms.

Exercise reduces cognitive decline. A study showed that the participants (aged 60 and up) exhibited fewer biomarkers of Alzheimer's upon engaging in 30 minutes of daily exercise.

Muscle power can be increased by engaging in strength training. One example is lifting weights. Day-to-day duties may become easier to meet after strength training. It can halt the decline of muscle strength brought on by illness as well as keep joints stable.

Stretching is one flexibility exercise that can help joints stay mobile to function correctly. Exercises that improve balance can help reduce the chance of falling.

2. Boosts the Immune System

Engaging in exercise brings a change in your white blood cells. WBCs are the body's immune system cells that battle diseases. These antibodies circulate more quickly, allowing them to detect diseases earlier.

A 2018 study connects moderate workouts to a lower incidence of acute respiratory diseases. There are many theories when it comes to exercise helping the immune system. Some scientific experts think exercise is anti-inflammatory, leading to better immune function.

3. Prevents Bone Loss

Age-related bone loss affects both males and females. Post-menopausal women lose up to 2% of bone mass a year.

Bone loss may affect your balance, increasing your risk of falls and accidents. But exercises can help you strengthen your bones, improving your quality of life.

4. Elevates Mood

Exercise promotes relaxation and fosters a general sense of health. It can even curb depression and anxiety.

A 2019 study of adult men aged 65 and beyond showed that exercise continues to positively affect mood long into old age. This data highlights how important it is to maintain an active lifestyle.

5. Improves Sleep Quality

Most seniors have difficulty getting adequate sleep. Sleep can be elusive, whether because of all the pain and discomfort of an illness or a general apprehension and stress.

For many people, exercise results in better sleep. Notably, adults who engage in moderate-to-vigorous exercise can improve the quality of their sleep by speeding up the process of falling asleep and sleeping longer at night. Additionally, engaging in physical exercise might lessen daytime sleepiness and, for some individuals, the need for sleep aids.

6. Maintains independence

Exercise makes you stronger, allowing you to take care of yourself better. While assisted living facilities are necessary for some people, it doesn't have to be required for you. Regular exercise helps you to maintain your living independence.

7. Aids in Cognitive Health

Regular exercise can reduce the risk of cognitive decline such as Dementia. Cognitive decline is widespread among inactive people. Moderate-intensity exercise is highly suggested.

8. Reduces depression and anxiety

Seniors experience illness, disability, and social withdrawal. All this can lead to mental health problems. By releasing feel-good endorphins, endogenous cannabinoids, and other natural brain chemicals, which help improve your sense of well-being, regular exercise helps reduce feelings of sadness and anxiety.

9. Assists in flexibility

Older individuals with osteoarthritis pain face profound challenges because their muscles and joints become tight and unmovable. Even though age-related joint changes cannot wholly be reversed with exercise, keeping your muscles and joints mobile is crucial for reducing pain.

10. Improves strength and vitality

If you don't exercise, your muscles can deteriorate. Like exercise increases flexibility, proper resistance activity enables you to preserve your independence by bolstering fundamental muscle groups. This training is beneficial when standing up from a sitting position, ascending and descending stairs, or simply walking.

11. Helps with weight loss

Poor diet and a sedentary lifestyle contribute to weight gain, especially in a person's later years. This weight issue results in a higher incidence of associated medical problems.

Exercise is a calorie-burning activity. So, you can expect weight loss when you engage in the proper routines.

12. Strengthens social connections

Exercise is highly fulfilling and holds you accountable when done in a group setting. Strengthening social ties is essential to maintain excellent health in later years, whether through an exercise class at the neighborhood recreation center or a regular stroll in the park with a buddy.

13. Increases confidence

Regular physical activities and training can enhance confidence, and this enhancement strengthens the mind-body link. In addition, improving one's self-esteem through exercise can promote satisfaction and joy and enhance one's quality of life later.

14. Builds a cornerstone habit

Behavioral scientists have demonstrated the habit of exercising to support other beneficial habits, such as wholesome eating and social engagement. Therefore, engaging in physical activity can have a variety of beneficial side effects.

15. Improves cardiovascular health

Workouts have tremendous preventative potential. Adults and senior citizens who engage in physical activity have a 35% lower risk of developing cardiovascular disease. Strokes and heart attacks are illnesses that can be fatal or have frequent and far-reaching side effects. Exercise can indeed be helpful in this regard.

16. Increases life span

If exercise helps you avoid dangerous illnesses, you should live longer. Research shows that regular bouts of exercise can add about three to five years to a person's life expectancy. Please note that exercise adds years to your life and enhances the quality of those extra years.

17. Enhances bone density

Osteoporosis, a disorder that affects many older persons, causes the bones to deteriorate and become more prone to fracture. It has been demonstrated that strength training, especially when done regularly, assists in keeping bones strong as we age.

18. Prevents falls

Falls become a severe risk when people lose flexibility, strength, and coordination. Illness or disability may also be additional risk factors. The risk of falls, accidents, and potential hospital admissions can be decreased by exercise.

19. It is a fun activity

Who wouldn't feel pumped up and joyful after engaging in exercise? Most people experience a psychological benefit from exercise through elevated dopamine levels, a brain chemical linked to emotions of motivation, pleasure, and well-being.

A Well-Rounded Exercise

You are now taking your first steps toward your health journey. The road to fitness is on the horizon. Are you feeling nervous? Are you excited?

Whatever you may be feeling right now, you need to ensure one thing - you have a well-rounded fitness plan. You need an exercise program that can promise and deliver effective results.

A well-rounded exercise program is composed of the following:

- Aerobic Training

- Strength Training

- Flexibility Training

- Balance Training

These four basic elements are vital in assisting those who are physically frail or need improvement in their functional capacity, and they are necessary for continuing and enhancing healthy aging.

Adding these four components ensures success in achieving your health goals. Let's look into each one deeper.

1. Aerobic Training

It is sometimes called "with oxygen" exercise. The primary purpose is to provide cardiovascular conditioning.

Your breaths control the amount of oxygen that makes it to the muscles, helping them move and burn fuel. The American Heart Association suggests a minimum of thirty minutes of cardiovascular training between 5 to 7 days weekly.

Apart from improved cardiovascular conditioning, the health benefits of aerobic exercise include the following:

- A decreased risk of heart ailments

- An increase in high-density level (good) cholesterol

- Lower or normal levels of blood pressure

- Better weight management

- Better weight loss results

- Improved lung function

- Controlled blood sugar levels

- Decreased resting heart rate

There are two types of aerobic exercise: lower impact and higher impact.

Here are examples of lower impact:

- Walking

- Swimming

- Rowing

- Cycling

The higher impact includes:

- Jumping rope

- Running

- Doing step aerobics or high-impact routines

2. Strength Training

As we age, our lean muscle mass diminishes. So this means our body fat percentage will increase.

But we can significantly slow this and, in many cases, reverse this through strength training exercises.

Strength training can help you maintain and improve your muscle mass.

Other positive effects of strength training include:

- Creates stronger and healthier bones

- Keeps chronic conditions at bay

- Lessens symptoms of chronic illnesses

- Enhances cognitive skills

- Controls depression

- Improves quality of life

3. Flexibility Training

It's all about stretching.

Flexibility training requires you to stretch your muscles. This movement helps your body stay flexible.

When you are flexible, you have more freedom of movement for your daily tasks and activities. Your movements are not limited or confined to one set of actions.

Your flexibility can also help prevent discomfort when confined in a space for quite some time. Examples of this are a long plane ride or a lengthy meeting.

Here are other benefits:

- Improved performance when engaging in physical activities

- Increased blood flow in your muscles

- More effective use of the muscles

- Lower risks of injuries

4. Balance Training

Everybody needs excellent balance to perform just about anything, such as tying their shoelaces, going up and down the stairs, walking, and getting out of a seat. Keeping yourself steady makes all the difference.

Balance training incorporates strength training exercises that help keep us in an upright position. These kinds of movements can aid you in stabilizing your body.

Other benefits include:

- Better body posture

- Improved body strength and vitality

- Lesser risks of falls and injuries

- Better mobility for stroke patients

- Reinforce self-efficacy in balance control.

- Increased walking speed

How Much Physical Exercise You Need

It's common knowledge that exercise is good for everyone. But when you are over 65 years, it becomes a necessity.

When you were younger, it seemed like there was not enough activity where you could burn off your overflowing energy. Nowadays, a little bit of exertion can tire you. Your energy levels are not what they used to be, and that's because the body has been more fragile.

But you still have to stay active. Staying put all day will only worsen your condition. You need to pump up and re-energize. Doctors recommend physical activity as part of senior care.

If you are 65 or older, engaging in moderate physical activity for at least 150 minutes per week is best. For example, you can walk briskly for 30 minutes daily, Monday to Friday.

You can also opt for 75 minutes a week of vigorous activity. So, you can choose 15 minutes of jogging daily, Monday to Friday.

Other recommendations are:

- At least two days each week, you should be devoted to muscle-building activities.

- You should employ balance-enhancing poses for three days (consecutive or not) each week. One example is standing on one foot.

Aim to be as physically active as your body and capabilities permit. If chronic conditions prevent you from making the above recommendations, you can find other ways.

You may choose low-impact exercises like swimming or riding a stationary bike. They will raise your heart rate without any pain.

You may also lower the weekly minutes. Even 50 to 60 minutes per week can be a big help.

Here are other tips you can consider when exercising with chronic conditions:

1. Instead of running - Walk!
It's much better to get off the sofa and exercise, even if you have a significant medical condition. Don't sit still all day.

Walking is one of the simplest activities that anyone can perform. You're not required to work up a sweat. All you have to do is get up and start moving.

2. Start slow and simple

Don't rush it if your health issues have prevented you from working out for a while. If your aim is 15 minutes per day, you can start for 5 minutes on the first day.

Go for simplicity. Don't go for complicated moves. They may tire you out quickly.

3. Use resistance bands

These bands are an excellent option instead of strenuous lifting. You can choose between mild, medium, or strong resistance options and change the amount of tightness in the band to change how challenging your exercises are.

Maintain proper posture, move gently, and maintain steady pressure on the flex band. In doing all this, you can get the best effects when using resistance bands.

Always consult your doctor before starting any workout program, especially if you have a chronic illness. They could recommend an exercise plan that meets your demands and avoids potential restrictions.

As you can see, based on the many benefits, regular exercise is one of the best things you can do for your health now that you are in your 60s or 70s. It can help you prevent or delay many health issues accompanying aging. Chronic illnesses, cognitive impairment, and bone loss are some of them.

But it goes beyond the physical. Engaging in exercise helps you maintain your hobbies and social connections. It can boost your confidence and alleviates depression and anxiety. The list is endless. All you need to do is engage in a few minutes of fun each day. Yes, exercise is fun!

You should focus on four essential components of exercise: strength training, aerobic, flexibility, and balance. While this book focuses primarily on strength training, it incorporates some elements of each component.

Even if you are suffering from limited mobility, there are exercises for you too.

Aging does come with health issues, but that does not mean you wait for those issues to come your way. There is a way for you to overpower them.

A healthier and happier you can happen. You only need to make healthy choices.

Hayley made the right choice. She chose to be healthy.

If she hadn't listened to Penelope, what condition would her health be in today? She would still be sulking during the holidays.

But she doesn't bother to reflect on that. What's important is that she chose to change the course of her life. What's important is that she lives a fulfilled life even at an advanced age.

Many others, like Hayley and Penelope, are living proof that it is always possible to make healthy lifestyle choices. These choices can be your saving grace, leading you to physical, mental, and emotional tranquility.

You can still make this stage of your life active and enjoy your independence. And while exercising regularly will help you achieve those, there is another essential aspect you should consider—nutrition.

Older adults have unique nutrition needs. But by pairing exercise with the right nutrition choices, you are well on your way to healthy aging.

Chapter 3
Proper Nutrition Slows Down the Aging Process

No matter how often Hayley has done this, the nervousness still prevails. With her heart beating quickly and her palms all sweaty, she waited anxiously at the lounge area of the doctor's clinic.

Hayley's least favorite day of the year has arrived. It is the day of her yearly doctor's consultation.

She kept looking at the grand clock on the wall. She kept glancing at the watch strapped neatly on her left wrist when she was not.

"Where is he?" Hayley kept muttering to herself. It seemed like she was waiting for hours on end. She has been in the clinic for a little over half an hour.

Who wouldn't be nervous? Hayley was about to learn the results of her medical lab tests.

Doctor Fraser finally came. Hayley quickly saw the smile on his face. "Could it be?"

She waited with bated breath.

"Hey, Hayley. Good job! Your results are exceptional!"

Hayley could not believe it at first. But the results say it all.

Blood sugar - Normal

Cholesterol - Normal

It's like getting an A + on a school essay.

But the results should not be a surprise, come to think of it.

Let's backtrack a bit.

Hayley is a certified sweet tooth. She loved chocolates, cakes, and ice cream. She can't wait for dessert every time.

Before her retirement, Hayley worked and traveled a lot. She needed more cooking time and relied heavily on canned, processed foods. With all the sweets and processed foods, and at her age, Hayley should have expected high blood sugar and cholesterol levels.

At first, she did not do anything about it. Then, she started to feel dizzy often. She had some unexplainable leg pain. In addition, she had an increased urge to pee and was always thirsty.

When she went in for some blood tests, she discovered that she had high cholesterol and high blood sugar. The doctor told her during her checkup, "If you have excessive cholesterol, fatty deposits may develop in your blood vessels. These accumulations thicken over time and reduce the amount of blood that flows through your arteries. These deposits can occasionally rupture suddenly, forming a clot that results in a heart attack or stroke."

Hyperglycemia, or having high blood glucose, means you have too much sugar in your blood. These excessive levels are due to the body not having enough insulin. Like diabetes, hyperglycemia causes rapid heartbeat, excessive hunger, vomiting, vision issues, and other alarming manifestations. If your hyperglycemia remains untreated, you can face severe health problems.

And so, the doctor advised her to watch what she eats. Hayley had to make some adjustments to her diet.

Whole meals like fresh fruits, vegetables, and lean cuts of meat are typically good for everyone. But they are ideal for those attempting to control their cholesterol and blood sugar levels. People with prediabetes and high cholesterol must reduce alcohol use and foods high in saturated fat and sugar. In addition, they must eat more whole foods.

It was hard at first to change her eating habits. But she had to do it for her health.

It all paid off. The results say it all.

At age 60, Hayley was able to improve her overall health.

Why You Should Keep An Eye On Nutrition

Have you noticed any changes in your appetite? Are you struggling to work up an appetite?

This situation is prevalent among older adults, especially seniors. They refuse to eat not because they don't want the food served to them. It's because they have lost their appetite.

You must eat well. Eating gives you the nutrients needed to stay strong and healthy. Therefore, loss of appetite is something that needs to be addressed.

First, let's look at some reasons seniors lose their appetites.

1. Losing the sense of taste

During aging, your taste buds lose their ability to detect flavors. What was once appetizing and delicious now becomes dull and bland.

2. Instances of Dehydration

When you are dehydrated, you feel weak. This condition makes it hard for you to do basic things like eat.

Most older adults are not getting sufficient fluids and get dehydrated more frequently.

3. Challenges with swallowing and chewing
4. Being sensitive to smells

As people get older, they become sensitive to many things. One of those is sensitivity to the smell of some foods. Some make them nauseous, making them stay away from the source.

5. Feelings of depression

One out of ten seniors is affected by depression. When there are feelings of despair, any thoughts on food are ignored. Some seniors also loathe mealtimes because they don't want to eat alone. Eating in solitude intensifies their loneliness.

6 . Loss of control

It's hard when you relinquish control of your life to other people. Most people do not want to rely on someone else to eat.

Because of certain illnesses, older adults may be prohibited from eating some foods. This situation makes them not want to eat at all.

All of these are reasonable causes. But no matter what the reason, you have to eat. Your body needs nutrients from foods to stay strong and healthy.

You can stay on top of your health by focusing on nutritious food and drinks.

Here are some specific benefits of healthy eating.

1. It helps in the management of your weight.

The risks linked with weight loss in seniors are occasionally disregarded since the risks associated with being overweight are given such heavy focus. Seniors who skip meals or consume non-nutritious foods might lose weight, and this is particularly true for those who use medications that include weight loss as a side effect.

Even though one must continue to follow the suggested weight-management standards, maintaining a healthy level of body fat may avoid rapid weight loss when ill.

2. It boosts your immune system

Our bodies use food to absorb vitamins and nutrients that fight off illness. For instance, most fruits and vegetables include antioxidants that protect the body from harmful free radicals.

Sugar causes the body's systems to become inflammatory, which can have adverse health effects and weaken the immune system. Give special attention to providing your body with nutrient-rich foods that will support your resilience.

3. It builds a healthy digestion

Older adults who don't follow a more nutritious eating pattern have a higher risk of developing digestive issues. For example, suppose you prefer high-fat foods, such as processed and dairy products. In that case, you are prone to experiencing chronic diarrhea. You are also most likely to feel nauseated or have stomach pain after overeating sugar or fat.

Since fat is difficult for the body to digest, overeating may upset the stomach. The colon may overproduce liquid due to excess fat, which could result in loose stools.

4. Improved cognitive function

Nutritious foods feed the brain appropriately, thereby improving cognition. The brain is like other body parts and types of muscles. It requires nutrients, such as healthy fats and proteins, to function. It is best to hydrate yourself constantly.

If you want to remain alert and intelligent in your older years, your diet should include healthy fats. Fat is essential for our brains to function, but it has to be the right kind.

You need to get sufficient omega 3-fatty acids. They are the essential building blocks of your brain and are great for memory enhancement.

Protein strengthens your focus. It's a necessary building block for brain health.

I'm sure you have heard of brain food. Here are some examples:

1. Leafy Greens such as kale, spinach, broccoli, and collards.
2. Nuts, most specifically walnuts
3. Berries
4. Fatty fish such as tuna and salmon

Healthy Eating for Seniors

As an older adult, you have unique nutrition needs. Making simple but remarkable adjustments to your eating habits is essential.

The meaning of healthy eating evolves as you age. For instance, your metabolism has changed now that you are older. It is less active than before. In this kind of situation, one needs to consume fewer calories.

With this change, you also need more of certain nutrients. This need illustrates the necessity to select food and drinks that can provide the ultimate nutritional value.

It's a good thing there is a lot of helpful information available for you. You can follow these tips to ensure you meet your nutrient needs.

1. Determine what a healthy plate means
My Plate. Have you heard about this concept?

It's an idea conceptualized by the USDA or The U.S. Department of Agriculture. It's an easy-to-follow food plan. Initially, this is meant to help parents plan to feed their children balanced and nutritious meals.

But it can be adapted for anyone. You can apply this concept to your nutritious eating habits.

The divided plate is separated into pieces for cereals, vegetables, fruits, and protein-rich foods. The interactive, user-friendly MyPlate website offers straightforward messaging to help you plan.

It states to pick a variety of balanced meals for many food categories. It also reminds us to make oatmeal, whole-wheat bread, and brown rice with at least half of the grains you provide.

Healthy eating is advised for any age group. But for seniors, this is especially important. Healthy eating ensures positive effects for you over time.

When choosing what to eat and drink, always keep those with the proper nutrients in mind. Your healthy plate ensures that every bite you take counts.

2. Be alert in looking for essential nutrients
You need various foods in different groups to obtain all the required nutrition. Imagine a rainbow-colored plate. Experts say bright and colorful foods are your best bet for keeping yourself healthy.

Lean proteins boost brain health, increase metabolic rate, and lower blood cholesterol. You can stay full and happy with a diet that includes protein.

It would be best to aim for many veggies and fruits; the best colors are red, orange, purple, and green. Essential vitamins, minerals, and plant compounds can be found in fruits and vegetables.

Include whole grains in your diet. Examples are brown rice and whole wheat pasta. Whole grains are particularly rich in Vitamin B, and bran from whole grains provides fiber.

It's better to opt for low-fat dairy. According to nutrition.org, the 2015–2020 dietary guidelines provided by the Dietary Guidelines for Americans specify the need to choose low-fat or fat-free dairy. This alternative is highly recommended as a part of a healthy dietary pattern.

Other reminders:

- Select foods high in fiber.

- Choose foods low in sodium.

- Include foods high in Vitamin D.

Vitamin D is an essential vitamin in the aging process.

3. Read and understand the nutritional labels

When buying packaged foods, always make it a point to read the label. Labels tell you if an item is higher or lower in sodium, added sugars, and fat.

Make it a point to review "Nutrition Facts" and the ingredient list. Some items may have false advertising.

It would be in your best interest to check calorie information. Far too many people believe that the label reading "110 calories" on a 20-ounce bottle of Coke means they are consuming 110 calories. That's far from the actual truth. In reality, you are consuming a whopping 275 calories; you must multiply the 110 calories by the total number of servings, which is 2.5.

4. Follow the recommended servings

You might find it difficult to determine how much to eat, especially since you have been advised to watch out for your health. Apart from consuming foods with proper nutrients, you also aim to consume the right amount.

There needs to be more clarity regarding serving and portion sizes. So, let's first find the distinction.

A typical portion of food, like a cup or an ounce, is called a "serving size." Serving sizes are not suggestions for how much of a specific dish to consume. However, they can be valuable when making food selections and comparing similar items while shopping.

The word "portion" refers to how much food is served to or consumed by a person. The size of a portion might change from meal to meal. For instance, you might serve yourself two little pancakes at home, while you might receive a stack of four at a restaurant.

Typically, the portion size is bigger than the serving size. For instance, when eating cereal, the serving size on the box is one cup, but when you pour the cereal into a bowl, you may have more because some bowls equal 1½ cups. So, you need to ensure you are following the specific recommendations.

What happens if you eat out? To maintain control of your portion sizes, you might try ordering smaller appetizers instead of an entrée as your meal. Another option is to share the entrée with your companion. If you don't have someone to share it with, you may eat half of the entrée and then bring the rest home to eat the following day.

5. Stretch your budget for food
Nothing is too expensive for healthy eating.

Understandably, some people find it hard to budget. However, there is available assistance.

SNAP or The Supplemental Nutrition Assistance Program can assist you. With this program's help, you can afford nutritious food.

Did you know that 4+ million older Americans use this program to procure food? The average senior gets about $113 each month. For more information, visit BenefitsCheckUp. org. You can check for yourself how SNAP can be beneficial for you.

Dietary Supplements

I'm sure you have heard about dietary supplements. But, like most people, there are certain vague areas. Since they are also recommended for healthy aging, let's clarify them.

Let's begin with the basics. Of course, it's best to define what dietary supplements are.

They are substances that can bring more nutrients into our diet. We take them to supplement healthy eating.

Dietary supplements contain enzymes, herbs and other plants, fiber, amino acids, vitamins, and minerals. When you take them, especially with meals, their suitable components are added to your food.

They come in powders, gel caps, extracts, liquids, pills, tablets, and capsules. There's no need for a doctor's prescription when buying dietary supplements.

You may ask why you need to take them. Isn't eating healthy foods enough?

Please know that some individuals don't get sufficient nutrients from their daily diet. It may be because of certain conditions. In such instances, physicians will likely recommend taking dietary supplements so that the person can still get the missing nutrients from their daily diet.

Here are some examples of nutritional supplements that are commonly taken.

1. Vitamin D

It is a fat-soluble vitamin known to help our body absorb and maintain calcium and phosphorus, essential in bone-building. Most people consume less than what is recommended for Vitamin D consumption. Using supplements can aid with that.

2. Calcium

Calcium is needed for bone strength. Older folks are prone to bone loss and fractures. You can get calcium from milk products and dark-green, leafy veggies.

3. Vitamin B6

It's a water-soluble vitamin that performs many functions in the body. One of the most important is making hemoglobin. Hemoglobin carries oxygen from the red blood cells to bodily tissues. Anemia is one of the most common outcomes of vitamin B6 deficiency. You can find this vitamin in potatoes, vegetables, fruit, fish, and organ meats.

4. Vitamin B12

This substance keeps the red blood cells and nerves strong and healthy. Some older individuals can't absorb Vitamin B12 from food consumption. If you are one of them, it's highly recommended that you take Vitamin B12 supplements. This vitamin can be found in potatoes, vegetables, fruit, fish, and organ meats.

5. Antioxidants

One dietary supplement that has been gaining ground is antioxidants. These supplements are top-rated and commonly touted as healthy. The reason for this is that antioxidants, the substance, are associated with many health benefits.

Antioxidants are molecules that may shield your cells from free radicals. Free radicals are typically linked to heart ailments, cancer, and other diseases. Free radicals are molecules formed when the body breaks down food when exposed to radiation, tobacco smoke, or both.

For your reference, here are the most common antioxidants that experts suggest to include in one's diet:

Beta-carotene

Veggies and fruits are abundant with beta-carotene, especially dark orange or garlic green ones.

Vitamin C

This vitamin is also called ascorbic acid and is a water-soluble nutrient. It helps prevent cell damage, making it an effective antioxidant. Vitamin C-rich foods include red peppers, strawberries, tomatoes, and all kinds of citrus fruits.

Selenium

Antioxidant properties of selenium aid in the breakdown of peroxides. Peroxides can harm DNA and tissues and cause inflammation and other health issues. Selenium is found in seafood, liver, grains, and meat.

Vitamin E

Tocopherols and tocotrienols are two of the eight compounds referred to as vitamin E. Most of vitamin E's advantages come from preventing a deficiency; however, there are a few circumstances in which supplements can be advantageous. Enhancing T-cell-mediated immune activity through supplementation with tocopherol strengthens the immune system.

Additionally, vitamin E appears to improve the body's immune system's response to immunizations. In particular, older adults need vitamin E since a shortage is linked to an increased risk of bone fractures.

Olive, peanut, and canola oil are rich in Vitamin E. You can also find it in wheat germ, sesame seeds, and nuts.

Herbal Supplements

Plant-derived dietary supplements are known as herbal supplements. You take these supplements orally, whether in powder, liquid, capsule, or tablet form.

Some examples include ginseng, ginkgo biloba, black cohosh, and echinacea. Researchers are investigating utilizing herbs to cure or prevent various health issues.

It's important to know that just because a supplement is natural or comes from plants doesn't necessarily mean it's safe to take, especially if you are on medications. Make sure that you talk with your physician so she can check for any drug interactions.

FDA, or The U.S. Food and Drug Administration, verifies the safety of prescription drugs, such as blood pressure drugs and antibiotics, and over-the-counter meds, such as pain relievers and cold medicines. However, the organization does not have the same authority over dietary supplements. Dietary supplements don't need to be FDA-approved.

The Importance of Hydration

Dehydration is harmful to people, whatever their age. However, seniors are at a greater risk.

Typically, the human body defends itself naturally from dehydration through thirst. When we feel thirsty, we drink.

But as a person ages, their thirst signal wanes. Even if the body needs water for replenishment, it does not realize it.

Aging affects bodily functions. Seniors tend to have kidney issues resulting in fluid imbalance. This situation eventually leads to dehydration.

The following are symptoms of dehydration:

- Less urine frequency

- Dark-colored urine

- Dizziness

- Arm and leg muscle cramps

- Headaches

- Fatigue

- Unexplained irritability

- Fast heartbeat

- Low blood pressure

- Dry skin and mouth

- Confusion

The National Academies of Sciences, Engineering, and Medicine recommend the following water consumption (approximately):

- 3.7 liters of fluid each day for men

- 2.7 liters of fluid each day for women

Here are some tips to stay hydrated at all times

1. Select foods that are high in water content.

Adding water-rich foods to your diet is a great way to hydrate, especially if you have issues with drinking fluids regularly. Have soups and broths; they are a great addition to your meals.

Watermelon, cucumbers, celery, and lettuce are great choices. They can increase your fluid intake and are so good to snack on!

2. Bring a bottle or tumbler of water wherever you go.

It is simple to occasionally sip on water if you constantly have it with you. Wherever you go, always have a refillable water bottle with you. Have a water pitcher available to monitor your fluid consumption if you are always at home.

3. Reduce your alcohol consumption.

The best way to dehydrate your body is with alcohol. As a diuretic, it makes you urinate more frequently, causing you to lose essential fluids. Additionally, alcohol depletes your body's supply of the minerals and electrolytes required to function.

Integrating hydration into your routine is vital. How can you do that? You can start your day with it.

Kick start your day with a glass of water. It will tell your body to get going. As your body is replenished, it will be easier to accommodate the fluids you will consume throughout the day.

Improving Sleep

Seniors tend to sleep and get up much earlier than what's typical. That's why they need help obtaining the required amount of sleep - seven to nine hours each night.

Here are some tips:

1. Follow a schedule.

Set a time for when to sleep and get up each day.

2. Don't nap.

They keep you alert at night, making it hard to get shut-eye.

3. Have a nighttime routine.

Spend some time unwinding before retiring for the night. Some people unwind by reading a book, taking a warm bath, or listening to calming music.

4. Avoid distractions.

Don't turn on the TV. Avoid gadget use.

5. Be mindful of bedroom temperature.

If you want to sleep better, the room must be at a comfortable temperature.

6. Don't eat large meals and drink coffee or alcohol late in the day.

7. Use dark lighting in the room at night.

One of seniors' most common sleep issues is insomnia--trouble falling asleep, staying asleep, or achieving good quality sleep.

You may use over-the-counter sleep aids if you have insomnia. But while these aids may be helpful, the effects are typically short-term. They cannot cure your insomnia. That's why having a healthy nighttime routine is good to have.

Other sleep conditions may require more than sleep pills or nighttime routines. Sleep apnea is one of them.

People with this condition often have short pauses in breathing as they sleep. If sleep apnea is not treated, it can lead to significant health issues like memory loss, stroke, and many others.

People's sleep patterns are frequently altered if they have Alzheimer's disease. People living with Alzheimer's can vary in their sleep patterns, with some sleeping more than others and others typically awakening in the middle of the night.

Always ask for your doctor's advice for sleep difficulties brought on by more severe conditions.

Hippocrates said that food should be our medicine. The road to good health starts by acknowledging the importance of good nutrition, especially at your age. Once you have understood and accepted the path to good nutrition, you can take the next steps. Always remember that healthy eating can do wonders for the body.

No one can better help you become healthy than yourself. Focusing on nutrition brings many benefits, like weight management and better cognitive function.

It's imperative that you now follow a healthy eating plan.

You need to be more knowledgeable about a healthy plate and nutrition labels to eat healthy. Healthy eating requires more than putting stuff into your mouth.

Nutrition is not only about food and drinks. It involves other healthy activities such as taking dietary supplements and getting adequate sleep.

Hayley focused a lot on her nutrition needs after her wake-up call. She decided to go on a healthier route. And look what that did to her.

Her latest lab results prove that making the smart decision to change one's lifestyle to a healthier one can only bring a person the utmost joy and accomplishment.

It wasn't easy; there were hurdles she had to overcome. But in the end, she came out as the winner.

Your road to healthy aging may also come with challenges. There may be times when the going gets rougher, but you need to plow on.

Your self-motivation will be your greatest ally. Motivation is like your car keys. It starts the engine that gets you going.

Chapter 4
Motivating Yourself

Hayley wakes up as if from a nightmare. But she did not have any.

But why is her heart beating so quickly? She sat up from her bed and stood up in a few seconds.

She saw the time as she turned on the lamp on her bedside table. It's almost 6 am, and it's time for -

Her heart leaped again.

And her eyes went to that dreaded piece of machinery on top of her dresser - the digital blood pressure monitor.

Ever since that ER visit, she has been monitoring her blood pressure.

"Check it first thing in the morning. Then, do one in the afternoon and another at night." That was her doctor's advice.

Hayley felt unusually tired a few weeks ago, although she had not done that much around the house. Then she suddenly developed a ringing in her ears. When she looked it up online, she learned about tinnitus.

She thought she could get by with all this. However, when she went grocery shopping one day, she experienced the most frightening dizzying spell ever. She fell on the fruit aisle. It's a good thing a fellow shopper was nearby, helped her up, and brought her to the hospital.

200/110.

That was the blood pressure reading. According to the nurse who assisted her, that reading is considered extreme hypertension. This level can lead to a heart attack, a stroke, an aneurysm, and many other dangerous situations.

Although the number went down, thanks to the blood pressure drugs given to her through an IV, it isn't over.

Her blood tests were normal, and her ECG ruled out heart conditions. What was wrong?

"You are overweight. In fact, you are a little bit on the obese side with your small frame." Her internist told her. "It's the primary reason you cannot normalize your blood pressure."

Then -

"You have to take measures to lose a lot of weight."

Hayley's heart sank. Dieting she can muster but exercise?

Her doctor proceeded to have a monologue on the benefits of exercise.

Blah. Blah. Blah.

She could not bring herself to listen. She could not imagine herself doing all the activities the doctor outlined to her.

She said to herself, "I'm 60 years old. I'm too old to be doing those things!"

And after a few weeks, she hasn't found the desire to start exercising. And so she hasn't seen any significant improvement in her hypertension.

She dreads using the monitor. Because she knows what the result will be. But she knows as well that she should do something.

"What's wrong with me?" She asks herself.

Then out of nowhere, she heard a voice inside her--One that sounded very much like her late husband's.

"The problem is, Hayley, you don't motivate yourself enough."

Myths About Activity and Aging

A big reason why most seniors don't bother engaging in physical activities is some of the myths surrounding fitness and exercise. Here are some of those preconceived notions and the actual truths:

Myth One
Exercise is no use. I will eventually get older and older.

Myth Buster
Regular exercise can make you feel and look younger. It prolongs your independence.

Also, continuous exercise reduces your risk of developing several diseases, such as heart disease, Dementia, and diabetes. Not to mention that the effects of exercise on your mood can last as long into your 70s or 80s as they did in your 20s or 30s.

Myth Two

Exercise puts me in a position where I can fall and hurt myself.

Myth Buster

It's quite the opposite. Regular exercise builds strength and stamina and prevents bone mass loss. Thus, you improve your balance, reducing your risk of falling and injuring yourself.

Myth Three

I'll never be the sportsperson I once was again, so why bother?

Myth Buster

As you age, your strength and performance levels will undoubtedly fall due to changes in metabolism, hormones, muscle mass, and bone density. But that doesn't mean you can't feel accomplished when you exercise, or your health will not improve.

The secret is to establish age-appropriate lifestyle goals. And remember that sedentary living has a considerably more significant negative impact on athletic performance than biological aging.

Myth Four

I'm too old to begin working out.

Myth Buster

It's never too late to start moving and enhancing your health. In actuality, older folks who start being physically and mentally active often exhibit more significant benefits than their younger counterparts.

If you haven't worked out in a while or haven't worked out at all, you won't suffer from the same sports injuries that frequent exercisers have in later life. In other words, since you have fewer miles on your clock, you will soon begin to benefit. Start slowly and progress from there.

Myth Five

I'm with a disability, so I can't exercise.

Myth Buster

There are alternatives. If you are confined to a chair, you undoubtedly encounter unique difficulties. But to extend your range of motion, build muscle tone and flexibility, and support cardiovascular health, you can lift small weights and stretch while sitting in a chair.

Myth Six

I'm constantly in pain; I am too frail.

Myth Buster

Exercising can increase your strength and self-confidence while also helping you manage pain. Many senior citizens discover that regular physical activity slows and reverses the natural loss of strength and vigor that comes with aging. Starting slow is crucial.

What if You Hate to Exercise?

Despite all the debunked myths, you may still be adamant about incorporating exercise into your life. You might even say you hate it.

But how can you hate something that could do you a world of good? Always think of the benefits.

Here are other suggestions to make it easier for you to exercise.

1. Find a workout pal. Pick a person whose company you genuinely enjoy.

2. Instead of chatting over tea or coffee, do it while jogging, running, or walking.

3. Walk your dog.

4. Watch a movie or a TV series while on an exercise bike or treadmill.

5. Listen to your favorite music while lifting weights.

6. Don't use a golf cart when on the course. Walk!

7. Walk laps at the mall as you window shop.

Staying Motivated

The most frequent excuses for not exercising are well-known to us all:

I'm too busy.

I'm too exhausted.

It's too dull.

And so on.

But there's one crucial factor - motivation or the lack thereof.

When injury, illness, or weather-related changes disrupt your routine and make it feel like you've lost ground, it's easy to become demotivated. But even when difficulties in life get in the way, there are strategies to pump yourself up and move toward your goals.

1. Focus on short-term goals.

Goals like weight loss, which can take longer to achieve, should not be your primary focus. Instead, concentrate on short-term objectives like boosting your mood and energy levels and decreasing stress.

2. Give yourself rewards

Whether you finish a workout, accomplish a new fitness goal, or show up on a day when you were tempted to cancel your exercise plans, treat yourself to something. Select some enjoyable activity you save for after working out, such as a hot bath or a cup of your preferred beverage.

3. Keep an exercise journal.

There are several creative apps you can use to track your progress. You may also go the traditional way - writing a journal of your goals and activities.

Such actions hold you accountable. There's a record, so you are propelled to take action. Besides, what you write serves as helpful reminders.

4. Find support.

When there is someone who knows what you are doing, that person has an understanding of what you are going through. They can be your rock. They can encourage you to keep pushing for your health goals.

How do you cope if there are breaks in your exercise routine? Find out what to do in these specific situations.

You are on vacation -

1. You can use the fitness center of the hotel you are staying at. Just make sure you pack your exercise equipment with you.

2. Do a walking tour. Only take the car or bus to go somewhere if you have to. Go on foot!

3. You can always do your routine in your room.

You are caring for a loved one, making it hard for you to find time -

1. Follow a taped or YouTube workout video when your loved one is napping.

2. Ask someone, a friend or a family member, to sub for you. You can go for a walk then.

You move to a neighborhood -

1. Canvas for nearby fitness and other recreational centers.

2. Look for the best parks or areas to take your walks.

3. Find out what activities are available for you to participate in.

You are ill or recovering from sickness for a few weeks -

1. Gather up your strength.

2. Return to your exercise routine after your recovery phase ends.

You are recovering from an injury.

1. Consult with your physical therapist or doctor on the best action.

2. Gradually ease your way into the routine.

Your workout buddy moves away -

1. Invite a friend to join you on your regular stroll.

2. Make an effort to connect with other senior citizens in your neighborhood; many are in similar situations.

3. Attend a fitness class at your area's community or senior center. Meeting other active folks in this way is quite beneficial.

Myths and misconceptions about exercise in your advancing years must be discarded. There are better reasons to step out of your comfort zone and be physically active.

Don't hate exercise. Embrace it.

It can raise your overall energy expenditure, which can help you maintain your energy balance and lose weight. Exercise reduces waist fat, which delays the onset of abdominal obesity.

Exercise does not have to be tedious. It is never dull. You can put variety in the ways to engage in physical activity.

Find your motivation. That's what Hayley did.

She took baby steps but steps nonetheless.

She has to keep going to see better results for her hypertension. She must stay motivated to achieve her weight loss goals. Let's talk about goals.

Your route to well-being must include fitness goals. Setting objectives can help you push through the most challenging times to make a change that will stay longer, hold yourself more accountable, and demonstrate to yourself what you are capable of.

Chapter 5
Goal Setting

Run continuously for 1 mile in 5 weeks.

Try a new exercise routine every other week.

Sleep before 8 pm.

Drink 8 to 10 glasses of water each day.

Take an average of 2500 steps per day.

These are some of the goal entries in Hayley's fitness journal. And they have helped her a lot in her health and wellness journey.

Penelope advised her to keep a journal for her goal setting since Hayley opted to do in-home workouts rather than go to the gym like her. So, the journal helps her stay on top of her goals.

As it produces a written record of her strategy and progress that she can refer to, journaling helps her define, establish, and track her objectives more successfully. Her goals and the reasons she set them may be more manageable for her to remember in the future.

The Importance of Goal Setting

For most people, they associate goal setting with work. It's a common theme in the workplace. However, you can apply it anywhere, including your health and wellness.

Setting objectives might help you concentrate your time and effort on the things that matter. It enables you to envision the kind of life you want to live. When working toward a specific goal, you frequently pay more attention to it and devise clever ways to get there.

The greatest motivator for you to keep exercising is to have fitness objectives. While long-term objectives keep your main objective in mind and push you to achieve more remarkable feats, short-term goals offer you a sense of an immediate target to concentrate on.

You can mark your accomplishments off the list as you go and set new objectives. You will find that accomplishing your health objectives will give you a fantastic sense of achievement, making you more driven. Your eye is already on your next target.

It's nice that you have decided to put your health first. But sometimes, you dive in feet first, riding the initial wave of inspiration. But after a few days or weeks, you lose motivation and give up.

A proven strategy is to set goals. Here are a few reasons why:

1. It keeps you on the right track.

You will have a far better chance of achieving your goals if you set them. That's obvious. You might be surprised to learn that many exercise or engage in other fitness-related activities without objectives or goals.

2. With goal setting, you can become more efficient.

By identifying a goal and the steps you need to take to accomplish it, it will be easier to meet it. That's because you have something you can refer to.

It's like having a grocery list where you cross out all the items you could buy. In your fitness journey, you won't find yourself stuck standing on the floor and not knowing how to begin your workout.

3. You can progress more quickly.

When you have clearly identified your goals, you visualize what's waiting for you at the end. You gain long-term perspective and immediate drive. It helps you focus your learning and better manage your time and resources. Before you know it, you are there.

4. You can get motivation from it.

Goal setting is an instrument of motivation. Goals do the following:

- Energize behavior

- Pose a challenge

- Provides direction

- Encourages thinking outside the box

- Devising new and novel ways of taking action.

Setting Physical Activity Goals

You won't get fit and healthy unless you get off that couch and start moving. How do you go about setting your exercise goals?

Here are some notes to guide you.

1. Identify your ultimate objective

Your ultimate goal is the most significant or challenging thing you desire to do. While an immediate goal is something that you're striving to do right now, the thing you wish to do in the end is your ultimate goal.

For instance, your immediate goal might be losing twenty pounds in eight weeks. Your ultimate goal is to live a long and fruitful life.

Sometimes, we get ahead of ourselves. We create goals here and there and lose track of where we are and what we are doing. So, it's best to put time and energy into coming up with goals.

In identifying your ultimate goal, here are some tips to consider:

A. Be realistic –
A realistic goal - what does that mean?

It is something that you can achieve, considering your knowledge and skills. You cannot expect to achieve the goal of winning the Olympics when you aren't into sports, right? A realistic goal also considers time and motivational level.

B. Be specific
Specificity means that your goals aren't broad or general. Instead, you should be able to pinpoint all the details. But don't go overboard; that might lead to over-complication.

Don't make your final aim a generic statement like

"I want to lose weight."

Create a metric for it. How many pounds do you aim to lose precisely?

"I want to lose twenty-five pounds."

C. Choose a meaningful goal
Pick a relevant and essential goal for you, not everyone else. Is losing weight something you genuinely want? Or are you trying to lose weight because your friends tell you you need to? It should always be about you.

2. Discover the ways to achieve your ultimate goal
Consider how you will get there once you have chosen your fitness and health objective.

Various approaches are needed for various fitness goals. For instance, you must routinely expend more calories than you ingest to lose weight. An efficient plan might include the following:

- Do some aerobic activities like walking.

- Avoid eating junk food.

- Have a smaller food intake.

- Dedicate 30 minutes of the day to exercise

- Consume more fruits and vegetables

- Choose lean meats, low-fat dairy, and wholegrain foods

3. Set small, time-bound goals

If you divide your main objective into smaller, more immediate mini-goals, you'll have a better chance of achieving it. Short-term goals are precise, regular behaviors or actions that move you closer to your long-term objective.

To efficiently choose both comfortable and realistic activities, you need to know where you are starting from. Then, you may progress steadily and at a reasonable speed.

Decide on an appropriate time frame. For instance, if your goal is to lose 20 pounds, a realistic weight loss rate of 1 pound of body fat every 1 to 2 weeks indicates you should give yourself 20 to 40 weeks to complete the task.

4. Measure your progress

Your mini-goals should be quantifiable. Have a plan for tracking your progress, and include every detail in a training journal. How can you do that?

First, you can use measurable metrics to gauge your progress. Consider writing down the weight and repetitions for each exercise if you are weight training. Keep note of your weight loss if you are exercising to lose weight.

Second, choose effective means to gauge your development. For instance, bathroom scales don't differentiate between fat and muscle. It could be preferable to measure yourself with a tape measure or look at how your clothing fits.

Third, take the time to discover many different ways to keep track of your progress, and do so frequently. For instance, if you exercise to lose weight, keep track of your workouts, daily dietary intake, and weekly measurements.

Fourth, celebrate successes, big or small.

5. Adjust your exercise to the changing environment.

Life is full of unforeseen circumstances. Prepare for them.

You can consider strategies for handling disruptions. For instance, while on vacation, you might not be able to exercise the way you usually do. What can be an alternative? You can always go for a stroll.

Keep working toward your fitness objectives, even if you are injured or ill. You can change the timeline for your ultimate goal. Create small goals to help you stay on track while you heal. For instance, you can still modify your diet even if you're too sick to exercise.

6. Don't be too hard on yourself

Yes, cut yourself some slack. Don't go for goals that may injure you in the process. Find a balance.

Keep a backup fitness objective in mind. For instance, being able to jog for 15 minutes can be your secondary goal if your primary objective is to shed 15 pounds. This secondary objective being accomplished is still a huge triumph.

Achieve Fitness Goals With Visualization

You can accomplish your fitness aspirations more quickly by using the practice of visualization. With this, your brainpower is needed.

What does it mean to visualize?

You use your imagination. You picture your dream in your thoughts. In reality, you're creating a clearer picture of where you want to go.

In essence, you're using all of your senses to imagine or reproduce an experience that causes bodily responses that are identical to really experiencing it. When that occurs, you are spurred to take action to turn that experience into reality.

For a more effective visualization, it's recommended that you start with something simple and familiar. Nothing is more straightforward than that.

Before engaging in visualization, focus on mindfulness or simple breathing. It will take little time--3 or 5 minutes daily will do.

Breathe. Relax—practice mindfulness.

When practicing mindfulness, you can tap into your breath. In and out.

Maintain focus on your task at hand. Is it jogging? Is it bike riding?

When visualizing, don't crush a single mindfulness or visualization activity. You can do short spots throughout your day—this practice results in consistency that will help you strengthen your skill.

Here are some things to consider when practicing visualization:

1. Get comfortable

You will not have it easy if you feel awkward or tense. Remember, you are only visualizing good things.

You can practice breath work 3 to 5 times a week. Each session can last only three minutes until you get to a point when there's no distraction and you feel right at home in what you are doing.

2. Don't be shy with details

Many details are essential in visualization. Don't limit yourself to the sense of sight. Visualize as well the sounds, the smells, and any other sensory information.

When you have vivid details, realism is more potent. Optimal visualization is like watching something in high definition.

3. Use positive affirmations

These affirmations are beneficial if you are encountering challenges with your goals. While visualizing going through a rough patch, say things like -

You got this!

Piece of cake!

There's nothing you can't do!

4. Crush negative thoughts

Sometimes, these thoughts pop out of nowhere. It's up to you to remove them. When you repeatedly rehash negative things in your head, it can be counterproductive. What's the point of visualization? Besides, these unpleasant thoughts can even lead to depression.

5. Be patient

A perfect visualization only occurs after a period of time. It takes time to enhance this skill, so don't get frustrated. Be patient and practice.

6. Try a beginner visualization technique.

In an article from wellandgood.com, author Liz Dupnick shares this technique from Dr. Eric Bean from the Association for Applied Sports Psychology.

Imagine exploring your house or apartment before going to the refrigerator and removing a lemon. Then go through the entire procedure of cutting the lemon in half, then quarters, before tasting a wedge.

This is a highly popular visualization exercise to develop your ability to use all your senses simultaneously, from seeing your surroundings to feeling the lemon's rind as you cut it to hearing the refrigerator open.

Overcoming Roadblocks

Every goal, task, or action taken will have its roadblocks. You fall; you get off-track.

For instance, you were doing well with your weight loss; you have lost a few pounds, but at one point, they start piling up again. Because of this, you get demotivated and give up. But you should not.

Here are some ways to get back on track.

1. Remember that you don't have to return to the starting line.

People think that if there's a problem, they will return to square one. That's a myth that needs to be debunked.

You make unstoppable progress; once you begin, there's no turning back. If there are roadblocks, you stop. But you only need to figure out how to move forward from the spot where you had to stop.

2. Think of the positive aspects.

Dwelling on negativity does not help. Instead of considering the roadblock a hindrance, consider it a stepping stone to develop strategies.

For example, you had to stop your daily workout sessions because you had to look after grandkids while their parents were on a business trip. Take that time to prepare.

It's an opportunity to learn. Take the time to research and create more effective techniques.

You can move forward quickly and more effectively when you are more prepared. Thanks to that extra time.

3. Prioritize

One of the main reasons we fall off track is when we subject ourselves to overloading. We must consider the time and energy needed to do these tasks efficiently. Sometimes, some goals need to be prioritized over others.

So, you must ask yourself - what is the most important thing for you right now? And at your age?

4. Make it sustainable

No matter what your goal is, make changes stick. When you restart, try to keep that in mind by following helpful advice:

A. Setting a schedule that you can stick to.

B. Enlisting the help of others to regularly check your progress and hold you accountable.

C. Starting smaller compared to the last time.

D. Being consistent with the actions taken.

E. Placing a greater focus on self-care includes getting sufficient rest, hydrating frequently, and relieving stress.

Goal Setting Worksheet

At the end of the book, you will see a sample worksheet. You can use it to begin setting your goals.

Whether work, personal, or health goals, you are assured of a better performance and outcome if you set your goals appropriately.

A simple statement of "I'm going to lose weight." is not enough. That's not the hard part. It comes with the follow-through.

Identifying and putting your physical fitness goals into motion takes much time and effort. But along the way, you can have help.

Achieving fitness goals has roadblocks, but you can take them in stride. Your visualization practices will help you do that.

Putting all this into paper gives you a clearer perspective. You can use the provided worksheet, or you can create your own. Like Hayley, you can have a journal. The important thing is you have something, a physical reminder of your objectives.

This physical reminder ensures that you can stay on track. You can always count on it to begin with your exercise regimen.

Chapter 6
Getting Started With Your Exercise Regimen

Hayley just received the notification. The equipment will be delivered today.

She asked a friend over to help set everything up. It may take time for her to get used to operating and using the stuff, but hopefully, she will get the hang of it quickly. After all, she has watched many YouTube videos that Penelope sent her.

She felt nervous but excited at the same time. She is now to embark on a new adventure that ensures a healthier and happier existence.

Required Equipment

Exercise is essential for the body's homeostasis and enhancing its fundamental processes. A healthy body and mind can be further ensured using well-maintained training equipment. Some that you may need are:

- Dumbbells

- Ankle weights

- Resistance bands

- Chair

- Mat

Although exercises can be performed without equipment, doing so has additional benefits for the body.

Just remember to start slowly and gradually raise the intensity as your body becomes used to it.

Of course, putting extra care into maintaining your exercise equipment is essential. Here are some ways to do so:

1. Clean it consistently

Hygiene is crucial; the equipment must be cleaned entirely after usage. Even at home, this holds true. A moist towel works best for all equipment, including dumbbells and treadmills.

2. Inspect it regularly

Regular equipment inspections aid in finding any weak places that may require replacement or repair. This is important for tiny components like loose bolts. By repairing them as soon as possible, you can reduce damage and prolong the life of the apparatus.

Physical Space

If you buy your fitness equipment, careful consideration is needed, especially regarding space.

Here are some specific considerations:

1. Space requirements

Your need for space will be strongly influenced by the kind of exercise you intend to conduct. Do you plan to do floor exercises? You only need a small surface area. But if you want to do lifting or buy cardio equipment, it would require a lot more room.

Choose a location with at least 6 feet x 6 feet of open space for the most safety and comfort. You'll be able to move from side to side and fully extend your arms. You can still work out even if you don't have a lot of room, to begin with. Make sure there aren't any obstructions in your path.

2. Optimum space

Are you planning to do your sessions inside the house?

Consider the areas of your home that see less traffic and may have practical elements already in place. As an illustration, the space at the bottom of a staircase can be large enough to do basic calisthenics, and the stairs can be used for cardio incline or decline push-ups.

Because no other spaces are accessible, many people use their bedrooms or living rooms as workout spaces.

Need more space inside the house?

A small deck or balcony can provide a great outdoor exercise space when the weather cooperates. Store equipment in a weather-proof bin to protect it from rain when not in use.

See if you can clear out an area of your garage as a dedicated gym. If your car (or cars) take up most of the space, see if you can come up with a small space to store equipment, and then when it is time to work out, pull one car out onto the driveway to open up an area for exercise.

3. Other considerations

Airflow

When selecting the ideal location for your home gym, pick somewhere with some airflow, like a window. You can put a fan in a small enclosed space, but if you work out and get sweaty and there isn't any airflow, your room can smell musty or shabby.

Ceiling height

Depending on the apparatus, a low ceiling can be an issue for tall or medium-height exercisers. It may restrict their motions, such as lifting weights over the head.

Make sure you can walk on the treadmill at its steepest inclination without colliding with the ceiling, if you use one.

Storage

Your choice of equipment may be influenced by how you store it. For instance, utilizing resistance bands rather than bulkier dumbbells may be wiser if you want to increase your strength by working out in your small bedroom because bands can be put under your bed.

Safety

If you live with kids, be sure you can store your equipment in a location where the kids can't get it. Many studies have been done on the possible risks to kids using mechanical exercise equipment like treadmills and exercise cycles, weight training equipment like dumbbells and weight plates, and even basic equipment like jump ropes unsupervised.

Now that you know all these considerations, you can get started.

Your workout area should be set up to look inviting and always available. Strive to maintain it neat and clutter-free. Consider decorating your training area to appear separated from the rest of the room if it is only a portion of the room rather than the entire space.

To identify the area as your "exercise zone," you might, for example, leave your dumbbells on the floor. You can also write motivational notes or a training regimen on the walls around you.

It's time to implement your workout regimen once your home gym is set up. It is helpful to arrange your workouts like you would schedule your attendance at your health club or in exercise programs. To hold yourself accountable, you might even want to enlist the aid of an exercise buddy.

Follow the manufacturer's directions to keep mechanical items, such as a treadmill or stationary cycle, clean and functioning if you have invested in them. You can clean other exercise equipment, like a mat, with a disinfectant wipe.

Proper Exercise Attire

Shoes and clothing are regarded as pieces of exercise equipment. Selecting the appropriate equipment is crucial for you for the following reasons:

1. Protection against possible injuries.

Some articles of clothing defend against collision, strain, and overheating. Compression clothing, which encourages blood flow and circulation to the heart muscle, is indicated for senior citizens.

2. For Endurance

The heart receives more blood when wearing high-quality compression clothing; the working muscles get enough oxygen. Controlling lactic acid accumulation, exercise-related weariness, and soreness are also reduced with proper clothing. All these elements help build body tolerance.

3. For comfort

The correct fabrics for exercise gear help lessen pain. Avoid wearing cotton shirts, for instance, as they absorb sweat and make one feel moist after exercising. Instead, use breathable, light materials to keep you dry and comfortable throughout the exercise.

Your clothing must give you freedom of movement. Choose lightweight, second-skin-like attire for your workouts. While performing a physical activity, it's crucial to avoid feeling constrained.

4. To prevent irritation

As you age, your skin becomes more sensitive. It can become easily irritated by workout attire made of poor-quality materials. As a result, during the exercise, you may develop rashes.

You may scratch yourself. Opt for lightweight, breathable workout attire to prevent skin irritations.

5. For confidence.

You can gain confidence while wearing the proper training attire and footwear, encouraging you to stick with your exercise regimen. Looking good and feeling good are closely related concepts.

So, what to wear exactly?

Experts recommend selecting leggings and pants that fit your height correctly. You might trip if there's excess fabric at the bottom of the pants. High-waisted pants may be more comfortable for older individuals since they do not cut into the tummy.

For tops, it is best to choose synthetic materials that wick sweat away, such as spandex, acrylic, nylon, or polyester. Avoid cotton since it traps sweat's moisture.

Growing older can increase the likelihood of overheating. So, choose shirts with venting or breathing panels for this purpose. Seniors who lift weights may prefer shirts without shoulder seams.

It's recommended that women wear sports bras for support. Please get one based on the level of exercise you will be doing.

For shoes - a single style won't fit everyone; therefore, it's crucial to try on the shoes and walk about in them. Everyone is unique in their body and foot shapes, walking gait, and preferences.

Before you begin

Before beginning your exercise journey, please consult your doctor or healthcare provider. You need to tell them if you have the following symptoms:

- Shortness of breath

- Dizziness

- Palpitations

- Chest pressure or pain

- Blood clots

- Sudden and Unexplained weight loss or gain

- Fever

- Muscle Aches

- Infection

- Foot or ankle sores that don't heal

- Joint swelling

You also need to inform if -

- You are having eye surgery or laser treatment You have a detached retina

- You have hernia

- You have had recent knee, back, or hip surgery

Technically, exercise is safe. But adhere to a few safety suggestions that can help prevent potential injuries.

1. Before starting any exercise program or if there are some concerns, don't hesitate to talk to the doctor or your healthcare provider.

2. Sharp pain-related activities, including those that cause joint pain, should be avoided.

3. Seek medical help if you have trouble breathing or have shortness of breath during or after exercise.

4. Seek medical help if you have chest pain or pressure and feel lightheaded and dizzy during or after exercise.

5. When feeling very tired or having severe discomfort, slow down.

6. Follow proper breathing during exercise.

   Don't hold your breath when exercising or straining, particularly if you have high blood pressure.

7. Build an exercise plan that works around your physical ability.

8. If not physically active in a long time, start slow. Build it up as you progress.

9. Utilize safe exercise equipment.

10. Unless medically advised otherwise, drink plenty of fluids, even when not thirsty.

11. Don't exercise outside during the hottest time of the day.

12. Do warm ups, especially those that increase the heart rate and loosen up your muscles, before stretching. Stretching your muscles without warm ups can result in injury.

Physical Activity Assessment

Not all exercise programs suit everyone, so please consult your physician and assess your fitness levels before starting any exercise program. If you have a history of knee, back or neck problems, you should use caution when starting an exercise program. If you feel discomfort, dizziness, or nausea at any time during exercise, you should immediately discontinue the exercise immediately and reassess your intensity level.

Chapter 7
Warm-Up & Stretching

"There, it's good to go!"

Hayley's son Anthony just finished placing her newly-delivered stationary bike by the corner in the garage.

"Wow, that looks quite good right there." She went by its side and looked straight ahead.

"The spot is just perfect." A window on the left side reveals her neatly-trimmed garden with a small pond in the middle. She can look at it while biking.

"What are you waiting for?" Her daughter, Eleanor, exclaimed. "Go for it."

Hayley laughed at her daughter's excitement. But she started guiding the couple out the door.

"Later, honey," she said. "I have to warm up first."

The Importance of Warming Up

"I'm already pressed for time as it is."

"I'm just squeezing some time in to do my stretches."

"I don't have time for warm-ups."

You might assume that skipping the warm-up isn't a big deal. But it is. Warming up before beginning any workout is a must.

You should always warm up before exercising because skipping it could have unpleasant and harmful consequences. Pain, muscle injuries, and strains are a few examples. In all honesty, a decent warm-up will really increase your workout performance.

Warm-ups (and cool downs) consist of lower-intensity exercises. They are done slower; with less intensity and pacing is just enough for a start.

Warm-ups prepare your body for exercise and improve performance. Cool downs, on the other hand, help your body recover from exercise.

Here are the specific benefits of warm-up exercises:

1. Faster Muscle Contraction/Relaxation –

Warm ups increases body temperature, enhancing nerve conduction and muscle metabolism. The outcome? Your muscles will work more quickly and effectively.

2. Prevention from injuries

By loosening your joints and increasing blood flow to your muscles, warming up helps you avoid injuries since your muscles are less likely to pull or twist during exercise. Stretching also helps in conditioning your muscles for the upcoming physical activity.

3. Increased blood flow

A few minutes of low-intensity activity can increase the amount of blood reaching your skeletal muscles, widening blood capillaries. One of the finest things you can do to prepare your muscles for a workout is to increase your blood flow since your blood transports the oxygen required for your muscles to perform.

4. Increased Oxygen Efficiency

When you exercise to warm up, your blood releases oxygen faster and at a greater temperature. When exercising, your muscles require more oxygen, so it's critical to increase the oxygen's availability through a warm-up activity.

5. Mental preparedness

When you go through the warming process, your mind will start paying more attention to your body and physical activity. Your training session will continue with this concentration, which will aid in developing your strategy, skill, and coordination.

Here are the benefits of Cooling Down after exercise

1. A means to recover

Lactic acid accumulates in your system after a vigorous workout, and it takes time for your body to get rid of it. Stretching and other cooling-down exercises can assist in releasing and removing lactic acid, hastening your body's post-workout recovery.

2. A reduction of DOMS

While muscle soreness is expected after exercise, a significant amount of DOMS (Delayed Onset Muscle Soreness) is very uncomfortable and can prevent you from exercising in the future. A California State University study showed that moderate-intensity cycling after doing strength exercises helped reduce DOMS. Cooling down helps to relieve excessive muscle soreness, maintaining comfort and permitting your body to recover before your next workout.

By not properly warming up and cooling down, you might suffer from the following:

1. Greater Injury Risk

Skeletal muscle injuries account for over 30% of cases seen in sports medicine clinics and are easily avoidable by warming up and stretching.

2. Blood Stagnation

Blood may start to gather in your lower body's extremities, which will lessen the pressure with which your blood can be pumped back to your heart and brain. You might have lightheadedness, dizziness, and even fainting as a result.

3. Increased Cardiovascular System Stress

By progressively raising your heart rate and breathing, you can better prepare for the demands of your workout by warming up. Your heart and lungs will experience unnecessary strain if you start an intense workout without first warming up.

Warm-ups and Cool downs are vital components of any workout regimen. Remember to add them to your routine for the best results.

Don't forget to stretch.

Stretching is one of the most basic exercises and one of the most recommended, especially for seniors. For many of them, being mobile might be challenging. As we age, our muscles and joints weaken, and our range of motion declines.

Let's look at how stretching can be beneficial:

1. Stretching eases arthritis and low back discomfort

Osteoarthritis is a prominent cause of lower back discomfort in older persons. The most prevalent type of arthritis, osteoarthritis, is brought on by the deterioration of the cartilage in the facet joints over time.

Usually, the accompanying low back discomfort is intermittent, but osteoarthritis may lead to sciatica (pain running from your lower back down your leg) over time. In addition to low back osteoarthritis, arthritis commonly manifests in the neck, fingers, toes, hips, and knees. According to Life Span Fitness, 12. 4 million (33.6%) individuals 65 and older have osteoarthritis.

Stretching exercises can be used to treat the ensuing pain. Seniors benefit from regular stretching by increasing their range of motion, suppleness, and flexibility to reduce stiffness in the affected joints. One could also use assisted stretching with a piece of stretching equipment or another person.

2. Stretching lowers the risk of falling.

For older adults, the danger of falling is a big worry. One in three senior citizens will fall every year, resulting in 2.5 million people needing emergency room care.

According to research, stretching is vital for maintaining stability and balance, which helps prevent falls. To reduce falls in older persons, increasing hip joint mobility and hamstring, quadriceps, and lower back flexibility is crucial.

3. Stretching can help improve poor posture

Our body's connective tissue, including ligaments and tendons, loses water as we age, making it less elastic and flexible. Poor posture develops over time due to the chest and shoulder's ligaments and tendons becoming tighter as a result of years spent slouching at a desk.

Consistent stretching is a simple way to increase flexibility. You will have more range of motion due to this helping to loosen tight ligaments, tendons, and muscles. Moreover, using senior strength training routines in addition to a stretching regimen will assist in balancing out weaker muscles and improve flexibility while correcting poor posture.

4. Stretching boosts vitality and blood flow.

Dynamic stretches will lengthen your muscles and improve blood flow and nutrition distribution. They increase the body's energy levels. Increased vitality is crucial for older persons to stay independent, stay connected to their social networks, and age healthily overall.

Safety Tips

Keep the following safety tips in mind:

1. Consult a medical expert.

Ask for advice on the most appropriate ways to stretch, especially if you have health concerns. There may be a need to adjust your stretching strategies if you have an injury or any chronic condition.

For instance, if you have a strained shoulder or any muscle, stretching may not help or even cause more harm. Also, be careful if you have a hip replacement. You may also want to verify with your doctor if you can engage in stretching exercises.

2. Warm up your muscles.

Do this before you do any stretching. If you don't, stretching may result in an injury. Warm-up routines, such as walking or moving your arms, can prepare your muscles for the upcoming routine.

3. Stop when in pain.

Typically, there's no pain when stretching. You only feel a little discomfort. So, when there's pain, something is wrong.

4. Don't over-exert yourself.

Practice slow and gentle stretches. Jerking and bouncing must be avoided because they can sometimes result in injury.

5. Avoid locking your joints.

A better way is to keep a little bend in your limb.

6. Aim for symmetry.

Concentrate on equal flexibility from side to side rather than aiming for the flexibility of a dancer or gymnast. Uneven flexibility on both sides could increase the chance of injury.

7. Concentrate on major muscle areas.

Focus your stretching on the key muscle groups in your lower back, neck, shoulders, calves, thighs, and hips. Don't forget to stretch both sides. Also, stretch the joints and muscles you use frequently or are involved in your activity.

8. Avoid bouncing.

Smoothly extend your muscles without bouncing. Stretching while bouncing might damage your muscles and make them tenser.

People frequently return from spending all day at a desk or a computer. Their muscles have had very little range of motion in this reduced position.

After that, they subject their muscles to strenuous exercise. Without a thorough warm-up, those shortened, muscles are vulnerable to injury.

What about after the exercise? You can't just stop. Give your body time to heal; allow it time to recover.

Each activity must begin with a warm-up and end with a cool down. That is if you want to avoid damage and safeguard your joints.

It might be challenging for many older persons to retain their mobility. As we age, our muscles and joints weaken, and our range of motion declines.

For a higher quality of life and healthy aging, stretching is something that you should consider incorporating into your routine. Benefits include:

The development and maintenance of strength.

Enhancing flexibility.

Increasing circulation and blood flow.

Of course, it's better to err on the side of caution. Take precautionary measures when engaging in stretching exercises.

Hayley knows her stuff. She knows what must be done before putting her body through all that activity. It's better to be safe than sorry.

Not all seniors are like Hayley, who still has command over her entire body. There are those who have limited mobility. So, it's best to know what activities suit such a situation.

THE
WORKOUT

Chapter 8
For Beginners With Limited Mobility

When Hayley decided to take up Penelope's advice on doing in-home workouts, she did some research. At her age, she had to take it slowly. She doesn't use a wheelchair, but since her retirement, Hayley has spent most of her time sitting down. She knew that she couldn't just go head first into exercising.

She read somewhere that she could start by doing some chair exercises. With appropriate movements, they enable you to warm up and increase strength at the same time. The movements collectively cover nearly every muscle group.

These can be carried out consecutively as a circuit. Hayley followed the suggestion of beginning by performing the entire set of exercises once daily for five to ten minutes at a time. She gradually increased the frequency and duration as she got more at ease.

Now, she has moved on beyond chair exercises. But they have helped her build a solid physical activity program foundation.

Chair exercises are beneficial for people who have limited mobility. They can also help those finding it difficult to maintain their balance.

When you do regular chair exercises, you reduce the risk of falling. The motions, though looking simple enough, can provide many benefits.

Here are some benefits:

1. They help with posture improvement
When you get older, you might do a lot of sitting. Your posture might shift as a result of this.

Regardless of your age, your body needs to maintain an appropriate posture. Your bottom tilts under, and your pelvis moves back when you sit. Your hips might not support the half top of your frame. Sitting also prevents your glutes and core, which support your spine, from getting any movement.

When this happens, the spine changes from its original S form to a lengthy C-curve. This slouch eventually interferes with your capacity to stand up straight. Exercising in a chair can help keep things from getting worse.

2. Chair exercises strengthen your shoulders.

It would be best to have strong shoulders even for basic tasks like opening a cupboard. But if you have decreased limb movements, the muscles will waste away.

Chair exercises involve upper body routines that can strengthen your shoulder muscles. Some simulate real-life lifting scenarios that can promote bone stabilization and better flexibility.

3. They aid in knee joint lubrication

Chair exercises are also applicable to the lower body. Some knee exercises can strengthen your joints, relieving you of arthritic pain, stiffness, and even swelling.

The Warm-Up

Here are some warm-up chair exercises you can try:

You can adjust your warm-up, stretching, and seated chair exercises according to your fitness level and health objectives. There are several options you can try. Just follow the steps to a T, and you are good to go.

The benefits of chair exercises are numerous. At-home chair exercises are a great low-impact way to integrate movement into your routine.

Now, it's time to level up. If you have moderate mobility, the next chapter is for you.

Aging-related changes might affect a person's mobility or capacity to move around. Mobility issues can include falling or having trouble getting in and out of a chair.

This chapter focuses on exercises for those of you who have moderate mobility. Moderate mobility means you can stand or lean on a chair for support.

The Warm up

Neck Turns (5 reps each turn)

1. Look up toward the ceiling. Then, point your head down towards the floor.

2. Turn your neck to the right and then do the same the left.

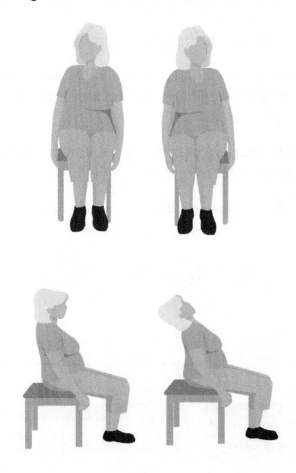

Tummy Twists (10 reps each side)

1. Put your feet firmly on the ground while sitting up straight. With your elbows at your sides and your forearms extended in front of you, hold your arms at a 90-degree angle. Then, rotate your body to the left.

2. Keep your lower body still and engage your core.

3. Return to the center and then rotate to the right.

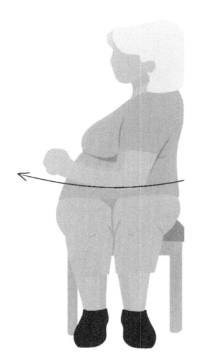 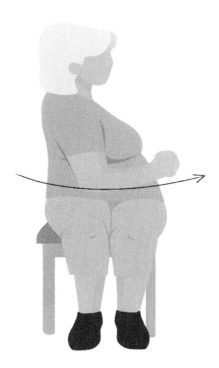

Knee lifts (10 reps each leg)

1. Position your feet flat and sit up straight. Lift your right knee toward your chest, then slowly bring it back to the floor.

2. Do the same with your left knee.

3. For a more significant challenge, pause for a five-count at the top of the exercise while you complete ten repetitions on each leg or twenty repetitions total.

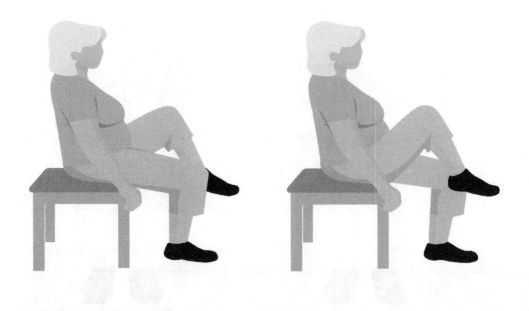

Stretching

Seated backbend (5 reps)

1. Sit on the edge of the chair as comfortably as you can, keeping your back upright and spine straight.

2. Plant your feet flatly on the floor. Ensure that your hips and lower body are in a stable position.

3. Position your hands on your hips.

4. Arch your back inward while your stomach pushes outward.

5. Extend the back until it reaches a comfortable stretch.

6. Stay in this posture for ten to twenty seconds, after which you release and go back to your starting position.

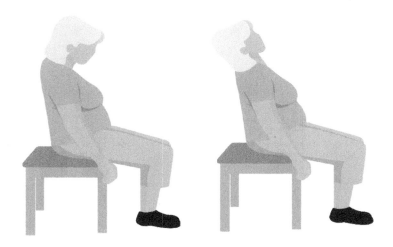

Seated hip stretch (5 reps each leg)

1. Sit back in a chair, maintaining a straight spine and an erect back.

2. Maintain a flat ground with both feet.

3. Create a triangle between the legs by crossing one over the other. Verify that the ankle of the crossed leg extends past the opposite leg.

4. Gently bend your upper body forward while maintaining a straight spine and a firm core. When you encounter resistance in your hips or glutes, stop.

5. Maintain the stretch for 10 to 20 seconds.

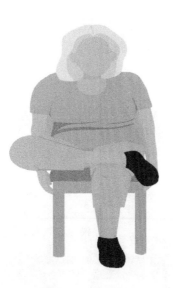
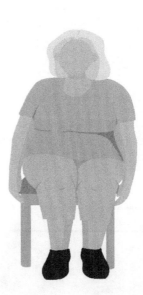

Seated Side Stretch (5 reps each side)

1. Sit on the chair's edge, maintaining a straight spine and an erect back.

2. Plant your feet firmly on the ground. To stabilize, hold onto the right side of the seat with your right hand.

3. Make the shape of a spoon or a prolonged "C" with the left hand extended above the head, and your body leaning towards the right.

4. Maintain the position for 10 to 20 seconds and then switch sides.

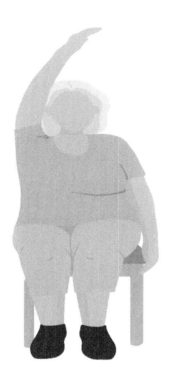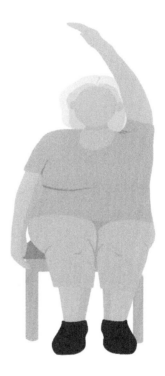

Seated overhead stretch (5 reps)

1. Position yourself comfortably on the chair's edge.

2. Plant your feet on the ground and put your hands on your hips.

3. Raise both hands slowly and connect them at the top of the head.

4. Stretch the abdomen by gently arching the back inward and pulling the stomach out.

5. Maintain the position for 10 to 20 seconds.

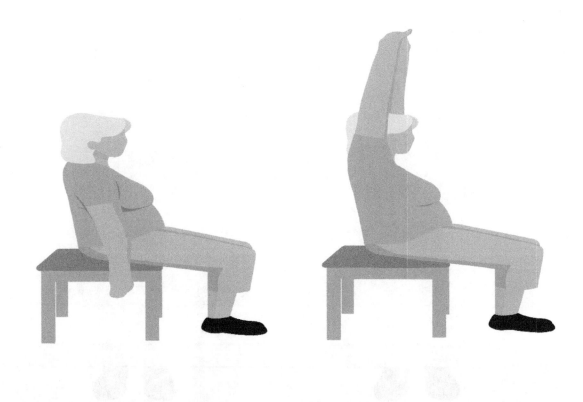

Upper back stretch (5 reps)

1. Sit in a firm chair.

2. With your arms about shoulder height, clasp your hands in front of you.

3. Drop your chin toward your chest.

4. Reach straight forward so you are rounding your upper back.

5. Hold for 15 to 30 seconds.

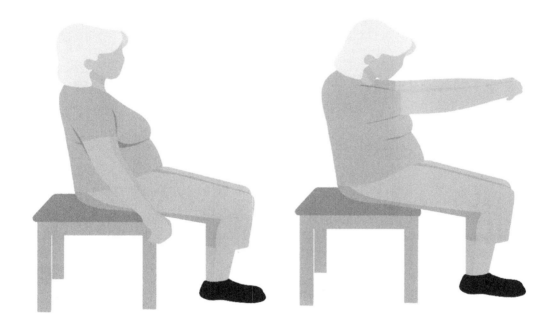

Spine twist (5 reps each side)

1. Sit to the side of a firm Chair.

2. Twist towards the right, placing your right hand on the back of the chair.

3. Hold for 15 to 20 seconds and then switch to the other side of the chair.

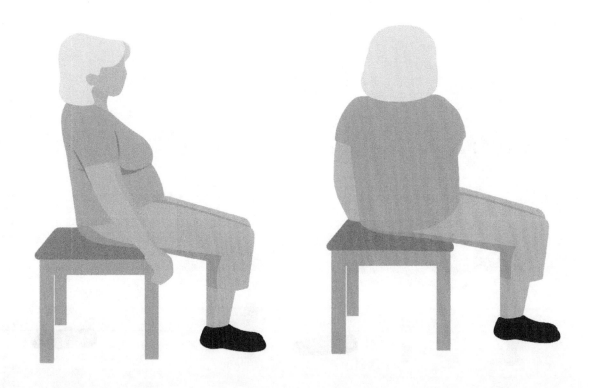

Chest stretch (3-5 reps)

1. Sit in a firm chair.

2. Clasp your hands behind your back with your elbow straight.

3. Slowly lift both arms at the same time, stretching your chest muscles.

4. Hold for 10 to 15 second and slowly return.

Tip. Don't perform this exercise if it increases your shoulder pain. Remember to breathe while holding the stretch.

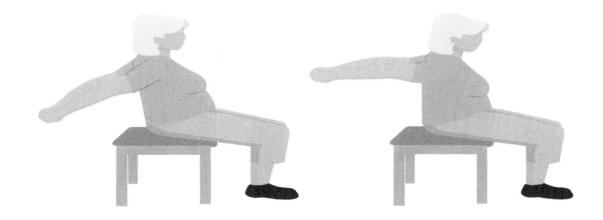

Back of thigh stretch (3- 5 reps each side)

1. Position yourself comfortably on the chair's edge.

2. Put one leg straight out in front of you with the heel planted and the foot flexed.

3. Bend forward at the hips slowly and gently while maintaining a straight back.

4. Repeat on other side.

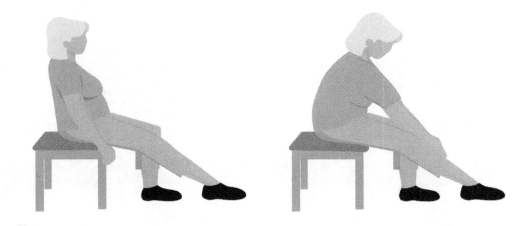

Knee to chest (3 to 5 each side)

1. Sit comfortably at the edge of a firm chair, with your back straight and feet flat on the floor.

2. Put your hands on either side of the chair.

3. Lift your right knee to your chest and hold for 10 seconds. Repeat with the other leg.

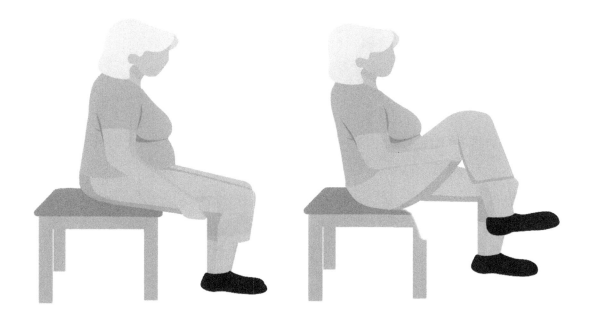

Ankle Rotations (3-5 each side)

1. Sit in a firm chair.

2. Rotate the ankle slowly in one direction for 5 rotations and then do the opposite side.

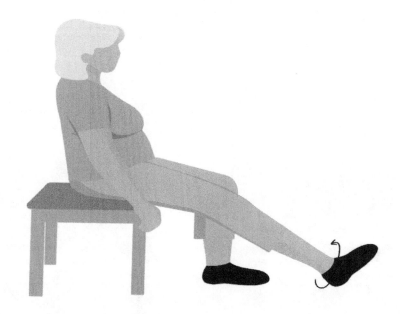

Seated Chair Exercises

Upper Body Exercises

Seated arm curls (10 reps) (2-3 sets)

1. Hold a one-pound weight in each hand.

2. Bend your arms at the elbow and raise toward your shoulder.

3. You may also alternate each arm.

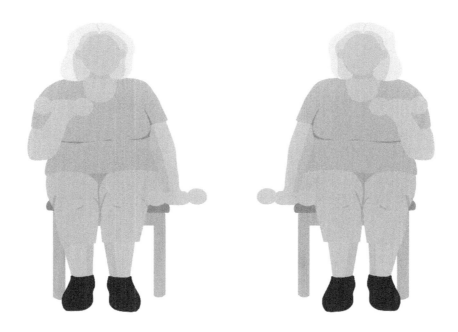

Bicep Curls with resistance band (10 reps) (2-3 sets)

1. Sit on a firm chair. Grab one end of the resistance band with each hand.

2. Secure the resistance band on the floor with both feet.

3. Pull the band toward your shoulders in a curling fashion.

4. Slowly release tension to return to the starting position and repeat.

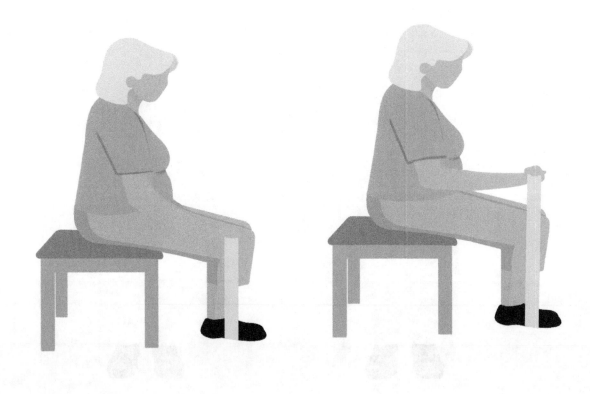

Seated row with resistance band (5-10 reps)(2-3 reps)

1. Sit on a firm chair. Grab one end of the resistance band with each hand.

2. Secure the resistance band on the floor with both feet.

3. Pull the band toward your waistline, while squeezing the shoulder blades.

4. Slowly release tension to return to the starting position and repeat.

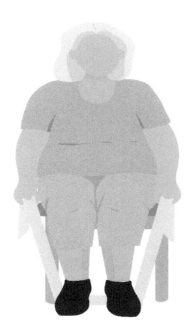 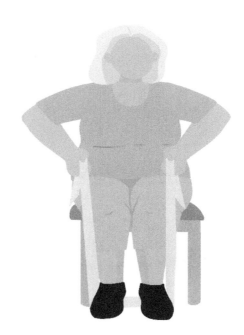

Banded chest press with resistance band (5-10 reps)(2-3 sets)

1. Sit in a firm chair.

2. Wrap the resistance band around the back of the chair.

3. Take one end of the band in each hand.

4. Hold the resistance band in front of your chest with both elbows bent.

5. As you exhale pull the band forward away from your chest, straightening your arms.

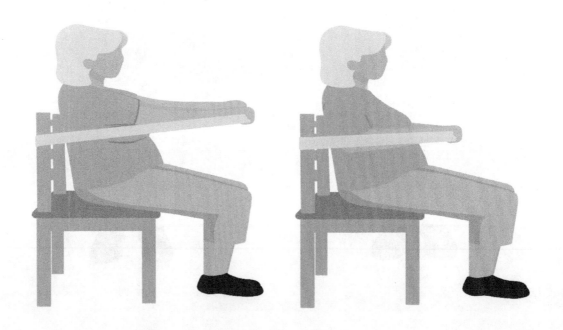

Bent over Row with resistance band (5-10 reps) (2-3 sets)

1. Sit on a firm chair. Secure the resistance band to the floor with both feet.

2. Grab one end of the resistance band with each hand.

3. Tighten your core to protect your lower back and bend your torso forward until your upper body is parallel to the floor.

4. Position your arms toward the ground.

5. Exhale and slowly pull the band upward. You should feel your shoulder blades drawing closer and your elbows are facing the ceiling.

6. Exhale and slowly release back to starting position.

Tip: You can move your feet wider to increase the intensity or move your feet closer to make it easier for you.

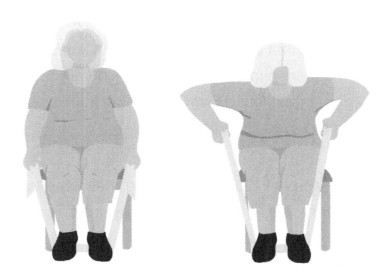

How Does It Feel to Walk that Little Further? Reach that Little Higher? And Sleep that Little Better?

"Strength. It does not come from doing what you can do. It comes from overcoming the things you once thought you could not do."

Unknown

You are just beginning this wonderful transformation, but even after a short time of making small changes to your lifestyle, you can feel the difference. The aches and pains that used to haunt your days are easing up and having more energy is allowing you to do more with your time.

The fact is, aging doesn't mean you have to live like an old person! Life after 60 should be fun, whether you have reached retirement or are looking forward to it, you now have time to do all the things you have never had the time to do. Nothing should stop you!

I have two hopes. The first is that as your physical health improves and that you continue to push yourself with some more challenging workouts you are about to discover. My second hope is that you share your new-found love for strength training with friends and family who could also benefit from improved fitness.

It's natural if you felt envious of older adults living their lives to the full without anything holding them back. It's very likely that others are now looking at you and wondering what your secret is.

Sharing your knowledge with others doesn't take anything away from you. On the contrary, doing a good deed for others only adds to your well-being. There is a simple way to help others who are in the same situation you were in.

By sharing your opinion on Amazon, other older adults can discover how to take back control of their health and live the best versions of their lives. It takes less time than making a coffee!

If you have ever read a review, you know how powerful these words can be. I want to be able to help as many seniors restore their physical health, but I need your help and the power of your words.

Scan the QR code below to give your review

Chair push-ups (7-10 reps)(2-3 sets)

1. Grip the arms of the chair and press down to push your buttocks up.

2. Lower yourself back into the chair. Repeat.

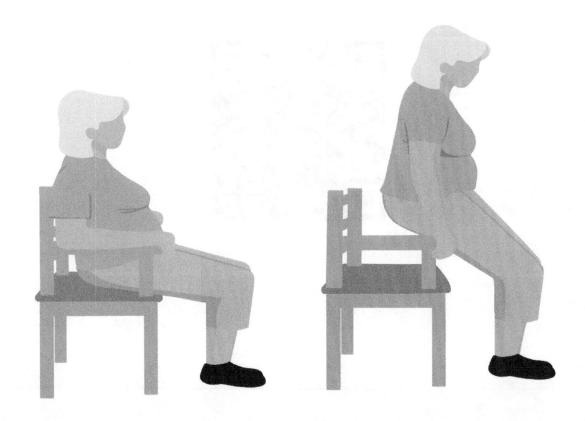

Lower Body Exercises

Toe taps (10 reps) (2-3 sets)

1. Put your feet firmly on the ground while sitting up straight.

2. Put your back on the floor and flex your toes upward.

3. Sit on the edge of your seat with your legs straight to make this exercise more challenging.

4. Ensure your heels are planted while bending your toes forward and downward.

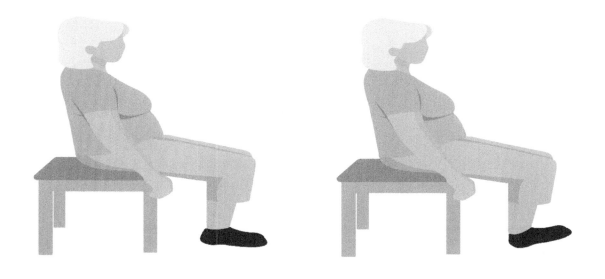

Tip: Toe taps help you strengthen the shin muscles and your calves. These muscles are needed to carry out daily tasks and climb stairs.

Extended leg raises (5-10 reps each leg) (2-3 sets)

Strengthening your core muscles, which can help avoid low back problems, is one of the benefits of leg lifts.

1. Sit yourself comfortably at the edge of the chair. Make sure that the position will not make you fall over.

2. Straighten your back and tighten your abs and lumbar—chest out.

3. Put your hands on either side of the chair. To keep yourself steady, tighten your grip.

4. Without shifting the body's center, raise one leg as high as it will (the ideal range ends at the hips). One leg will remain in the beginning position.

5. Repeat with the other leg, lowering it gradually back to its starting position.

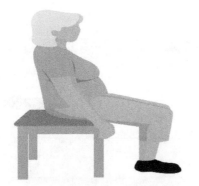 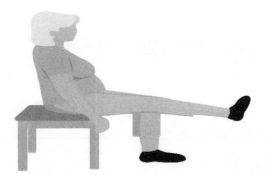

Seated Hip Marching (5-10 reps) (2-3 sets)

1. Sit fully back into your chair with your back straight.

2. Alternate lifting legs up and down, as if you are marching up and down stairs.

3. Rest for about 30 seconds and repeat the exercise again.

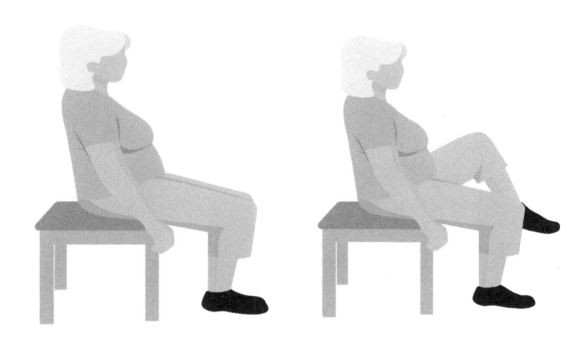

If you are pretty mobile but still have some movement issues, don't worry. There are multiple ways for you to warm up, stretch, and exercise with minimal motion. The list above is a great stop, but you can check out a few more if you want some variety in your workout.

Chair workouts are an excellent activity for seniors, and you don't need complicated machinery or a personal trainer.

The only equipment you need is a chair. Some exercises above may need a resistance band or dumbbells to be done correctly and effectively.

Of course, there are more than chair routines. If your health and mobility allow, you can move to other activities.

No worries, though. The next chapter covers various activities that improve balance, flexibility, and strength without compromising safety.

Chapter 9
For Beginners with Moderate Ability

The Warm Up

Calf Raises (10 reps)

1. Stand up nice and tall beside your chair.

2. While holding on to it, come up on your toes.

3. Hold it. Then come down on those toes.

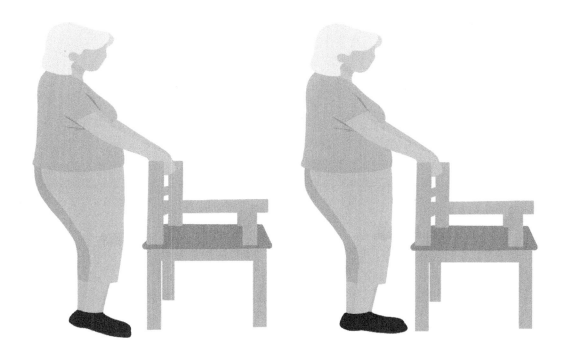

Ankle Circles (5 reps for each foot)

1. In the same standing position, lift one foot slightly.

2. Rotate it to one side three to four times.

3. Rotate it to the other side three to four times.

4. Put your foot down and do the other side.

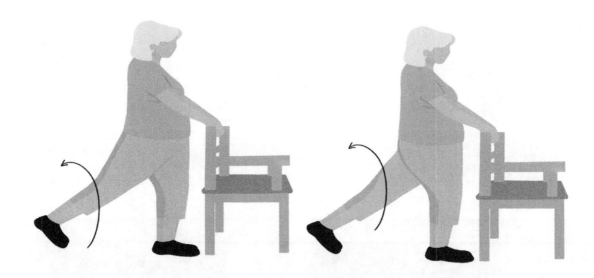

Hip circles (5-10 reps)

1. Stand still and put your hands on your hips.

2. Move the hips in a circular motion, counting from one to three.

3. Then make the circular motion toward the other side, exact count.

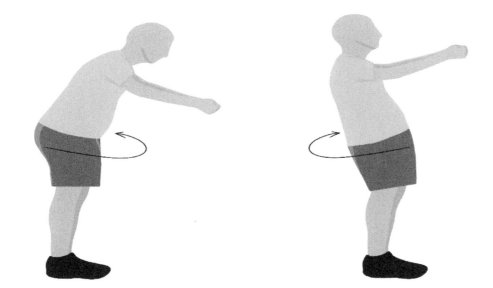

(See Stretching exercises for Beginners)

Upper Body Exercises

Chest Pull with resistance band (5-10 reps) (2-3 sets)

1. Grasp both ends of your resistance band. This position should be in front of your chest with your elbows bent. If your resistance band is too long, you can fold it in half before starting.

2. Exhale and pull the band as you bring it closer to your chest and try to straighten your arms.

3. Return to starting position

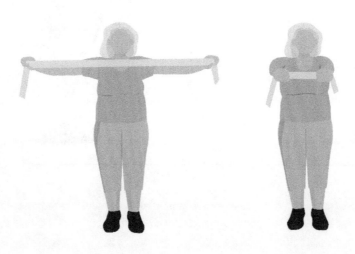

Tip: This exercise can be done while seated or standing.

Lateral Raise with resistance band (5-10 reps) (2-3 sets)

1. While standing, step on the middle of your resistance band with both feet flat on the floor.

2. Grip both handles of your band.

3. Raise both arms to the side, at the height of your shoulder and then return to starting position.

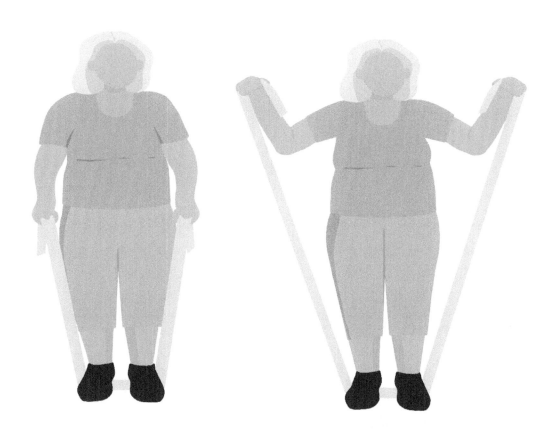

Band Triceps Pull with resistance band
(5-10 reps each side) (2-3 sets)

1. While standing, place the resistance band under your right heel.

2. Hold the other end of the band with both hands and stretch it so you hold both ends behind your right ear.

3. Pull it above your head and then release it back behind your ears.

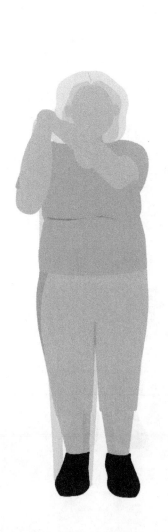
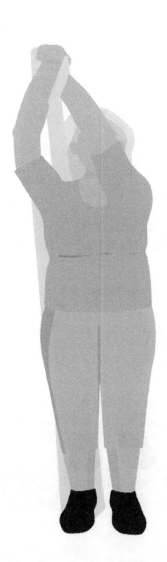

Wall Push ups (5-7 reps) (2-3 sets)

1. From the starting position, with you leaning forward with straight arms and your palms flat against the wall

2. Pause for one or two seconds at the top of the movement before moving on to the next step.

3. Exhale while you push yourself away from the wall with the slow and controlled straightening of your arms. Do this to a count of two.

4. One rep of the push-up is complete when you are back in the starting position, making sure you don't lock your elbows

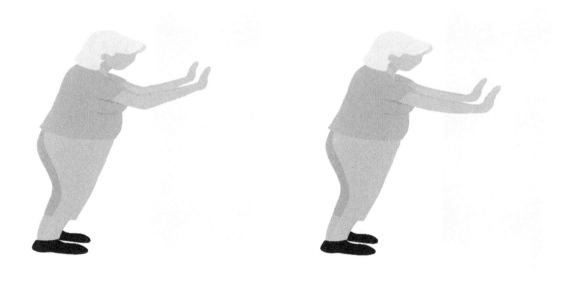

Tip: All the movements of wall push-ups, and any other push-up variation, must be slow and controlled. Lowering yourself too quickly and uncontrolled could cause you to lose your balance, yet moving too slowly could tire you out very quickly.

Bicep curl with resistance band (5-10 reps) (2-3 sets)

1. Step on the middle of your resistance band. Your feet should be flat on the floor.

2. Grip both ends with your hands.

3. Raise your arms to the height of your chest in front of you and then return to staring position.

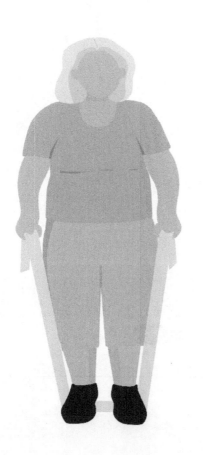 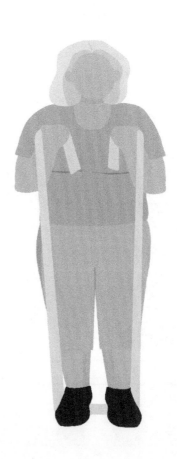

Lower Body Exercises

Partial Squats (5-10 reps) (2-3 sets)

1. Hold on to the back of the chair.

2. Sit back in a partial squat.

3. Return to the starting position

4. Try to go down slightly deeper

5. Return to the starting position and repeat

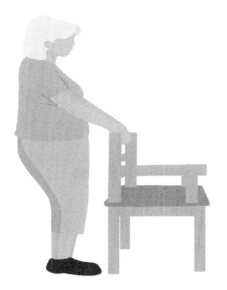 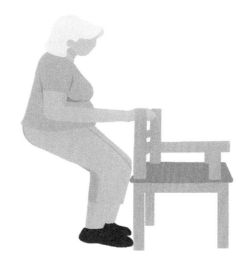

Chair Lunges (5-10 reps each leg) (2-3 sets)

1. Stand with one foot about 3 feet in front of the other.

2. Hold a chair or some railing for balance.

3. Keep your upper torso straight, and bend your knees and legs forward toward the floor.

4. Do not let your knee, which is in the front, bend over your toe.

5. Push back through your front heel to come up again.

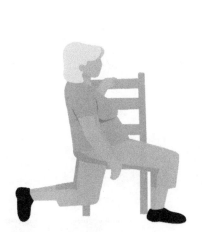
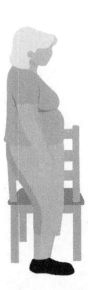

Sit and Stand Squats (5-10 reps) (2-3 sets)

1. Start seated in a firm chair, feet planted on the floor about hip-distance apart.

2. Engage your core and tilt forward from the hips with little help from your hands or arms.

3. Push your weight through all four corners of your feet and push yourself to stand, stretching your knees and hips fully.

4. Change the motion, gently bending the knees and lowering yourself to a sitting pose.

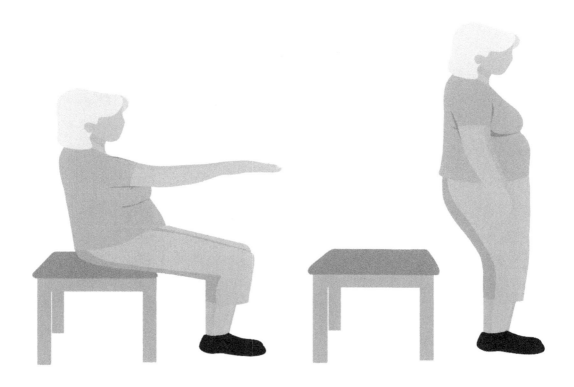

Leg extensions (5-10 reps) (2-3 sets)

1. Sit in a chair without armrests. The small of your back must be pressed firmly by the back of the chair, and your body must be straight and your shoulders back.

2. Look forward with your chin up. Your feet must be flat on the ground, shoulder-width apart.

3. Using ankle weights secured firmly to each of your ankles, hold the chair with both hands. But don't grip too tightly.

4. Inhale and exhale as you carefully straighten one of your legs. Please do not lock your knee into place; maintain contact between your lower back and the back of the chair.

5. Hold the pose for a second. Slowly, you should return to your initial position. Inhale as you return.

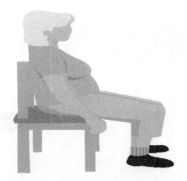 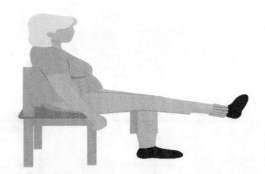

Standing hamstring curl (5-10 reps) (2-3 sets)

1. Stand with your feet hip-width apart. Place your hands on your waist or on a chair for balance.

2. Slowly bend your right knee, bringing your heel toward your butt. Keep your thighs parallel.

3. Slowly lower your foot.

4. Repeat with the other leg.

Tip: You may use ankle weights, if desired.

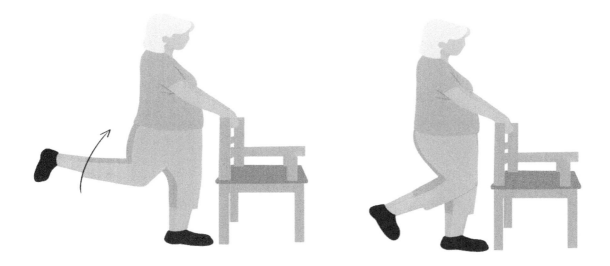

Seated Leg Extension with Resistance Band (10 reps) (2-3 sets)

1. Sit on the edge of a chair or bench, feet flat and back straight.

2. Place one end of the resistance band either under your left foot or wrapped around the rear left chair leg.

3. Make a loop at the opposite end and place it around your right ankle.

4. Grasp sides of chair with your hands for support or put on your lap.

5. EXHALE: Straighten right knee until fully extended (parallel to floor) but not locked.

6. INHALE: Bend knee to return to starting position to complete one rep.

7. Finish all reps on one leg and then switch sides.

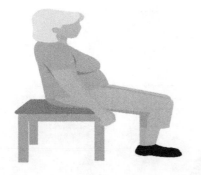
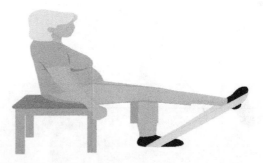

Modified Burpees (5-10 reps) (2-3 sets)

1. Get a chair and push it up against a wall with the back against it.

2. Standing with your feet roughly shoulder-width apart, face the chair.

3. To get into a half-squat position, push your hips back and flex your knees.

4. With your arms fully extended and palms facing inward, firmly place both hands on the chair's seat.

5. Step one foot back, then the other, forming a modified chair plank position with your body aligned in a straight line from heels to head.

6. Reverse the motion, then advance each foot to the beginning position.

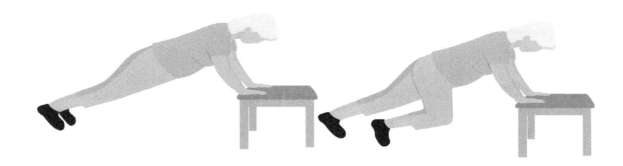

Modified Chair Plank

1. Stand in front of a sturdy chair

2. Place your forearms on the seat.

3. Step your feet back into a plank position and hold for 10 to 60 seconds (whatever you can do).

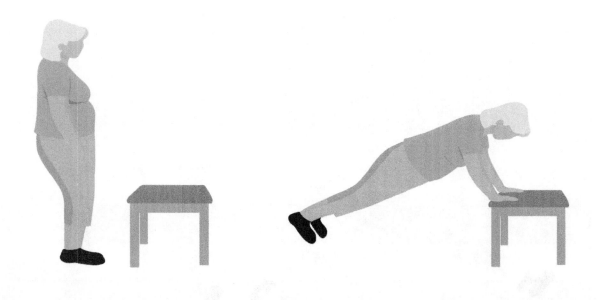

Chapter 10
Intermediate Work Out

People have different levels of comfort and confidence when it comes to exercising. But if you are ready to take it to the next level, then pay attention. The following recommendations are mainly designed to improve your flexibility and strength.

You'll have improved blood circulation and more muscle in the areas that support your body due to exercises that increase flexibility, which helps ease movement. Also, good posture minimizes pressure on your spine and core muscles, lessening pain from linked conditions.

Participating in regular strengthening activities, which assist in preventing osteoporosis and frailty by encouraging the growth of muscle and bone, is crucial to maintaining strength and vitality as you age. Having a solid physical self helps with both mental and emotional well-being.

You may perform dozens of workouts to increase your strength and flexibility without setting foot inside a gym. For those just starting, here are a few examples.

The Warm Up

It is essential to warm up. Doing so dilates your blood vessels, enabling oxygen supply to your muscles. A warm-up also slowly raises your heart's pace to lessen the stress. Jogging in place is a great way to start; you can do this for one minute.

Here are additional ones. Go through the following warm-up moves for about one minute each. Do not rest between each movement, but take a few seconds if needed.

Stretching

There are two distinct kinds of stretches:

1. Static
They often entail contracting specific muscles and holding the stretch for a few seconds. Nevertheless, if you have yet to warm up, this won't benefit your muscles. Save the static stretches for your cool down after your workout.

2. Dynamic

They are beneficial to perform as part of your warm-up before a workout. Dynamic stretches involve a variety of actions to stimulate your joints and muscles. It can entail imitating your movements from the sport or activity you're warming up for, but less vigorously.

Dynamic stretches will help you maintain fitness while enhancing joint and muscle health. They are a great companion to a nutritious diet.

Here are some dynamic stretches you can try. Let's begin with some core and lower body dynamic stretches.

The warm up

Basic Squats (5-10 reps)

1. Put your feet hip-distance apart and stand tall. Your toes, knees, and hips ought to be pointed forward. As if you were going to recline back onto a chair.

2. Flex your knees and extend your buttocks rearward.

3. Keep your weight on your heels and your knees on your toes at all times. Rise once and then slowly return to the squat position.

Tip: Try to bring your glutes as low as possible.

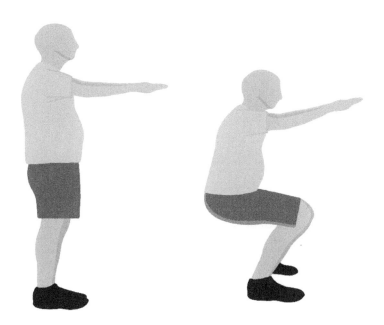

- Jog in place for 60 seconds.

- March with high knees for 60 seconds.

Stretching

Standing squat stretch (5 to 10 reps)

1. Place your feet shoulder-width apart while standing up straight. Switch to using one leg for balance.

2. Take hold of the opposing ankle with your opposite hand and bring it toward your butt.

4. Keep your hips moving forward and your chest out as you stretch.

5. Hold the position for around 20 seconds.

6. Do the other side

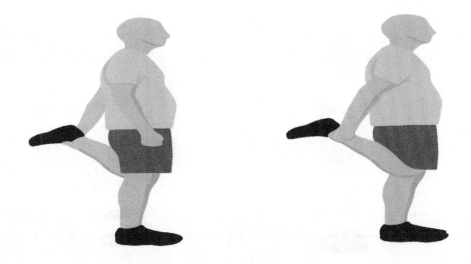

Tip: If you have trouble maintaining your equilibrium, take a seat close to a wall or other sturdy object.

Hula hoop hip stretches (5-10 rotations)

1. Set your feet firmly together and stand straight up.

2. Your hands should be on your hips. Imagine twirling a hula hoop around your waist while you rotate your hips.

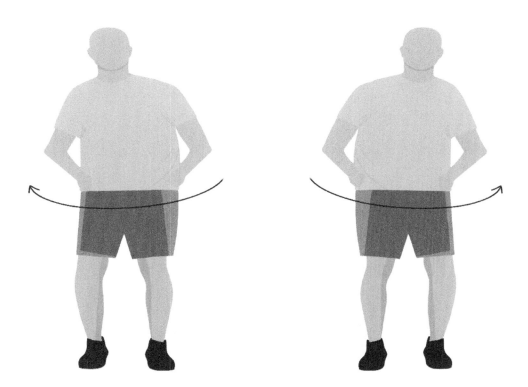

Shoulder stretch (5 reps each side)

1. While supporting yourself with your opposite hand, bring one arm over your chest.

2. Try to raise your inner elbow up to your chest as much as you can. Maintain the posture for 10 to 15 seconds.

3. Do the opposite side

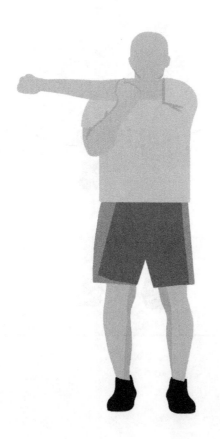 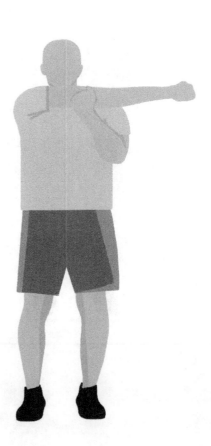

Chin drop (5-7 reps)

1. Set your feet firmly together and stand straight up.

2. Drop you chin towards your chest and hold for 5 seconds.

3. Bring your chip up to the resting posture.

Tip: You can do this standing or seated.

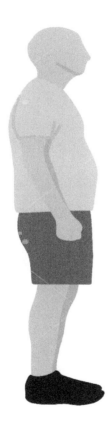 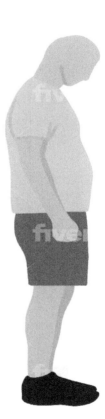

Arm opener (5-7 reps)

1. Place your feet shoulder-width apart while standing up straight.

2. Cross your arms across your chest. Open your arms as wide as you can. And hold for 20 seconds.

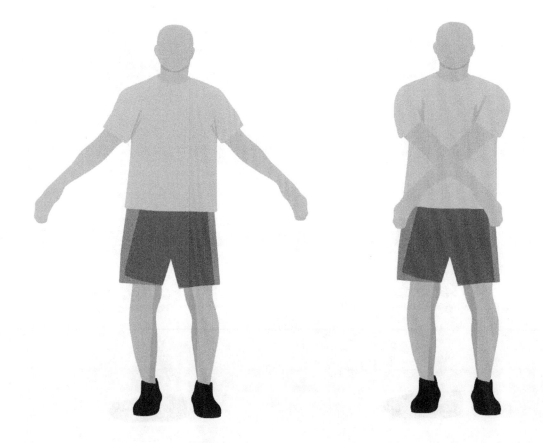

Double-knee torso rotation (5-7 reps)

1. Lay down on your back. Put your feet level on the ground while bending your knees. Form a T with your arms by spreading them widely.

2. As you raise both knees toward your chest, keep your abs tight. When lowering your head to the other side, sag your legs to one side and keep your arms at your sides.

3. Maintain the posture and slowly bring your knees back to the middle before repeating the movement, this time moving toward the opposing side.

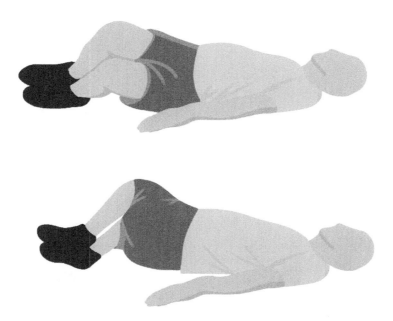

Upper Body Exercises

Shoulder Overhead Press (10-12 rep) (2-3 sets)

1. Stand upright and keep the back straight. Hold a dumbbell in each hand, at the shoulders, with an overhand grip. Thumbs are on the inside and knuckles face up.

2. Exhale as you raise the weights above the head in a controlled motion.

3. Pause briefly at the top of the motion.

4. Inhale and return the dumbbells to the shoulders.

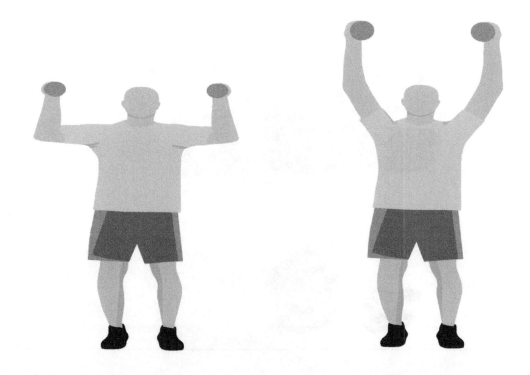

Shoulder Shrugs (10-12 reps) (2-3 sets)

1. Keep your chin up, facing straight ahead, and your neck straight.

2. While you inhale, bring your shoulders as high up toward your ears as you can.

3. Do the movement slowly so that you feel the resistance of your muscles.

4. Lower your shoulders back down and breathe out before repeating the movement

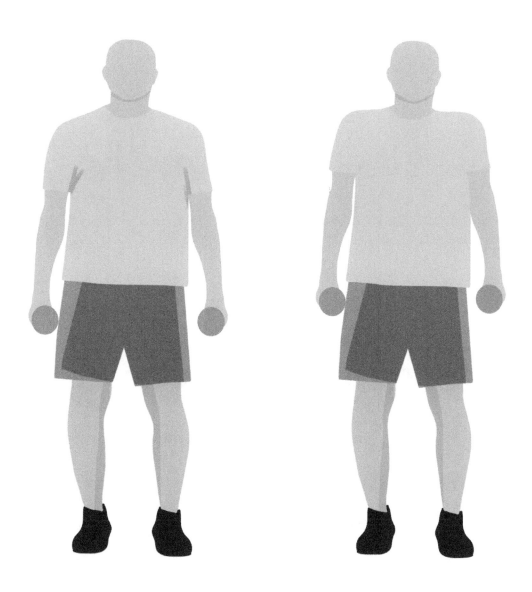

Dumbbell Curl (10-12 reps) (2-3 sets)

1. Start by standing up in a good posture with a dumbbell in each hand, squeezing the handle of the dumbbell as hard as possible.

2. Hinge forward very slightly at your hips and take a breath in.

3. Breathing out, start to curl the dumbbell up, then about half way up, twist (or supinate) your hand so your pinky finger twists towards your face.

4. At the top of the movement, contract your bicep as much as possible, getting a good peak squeeze.

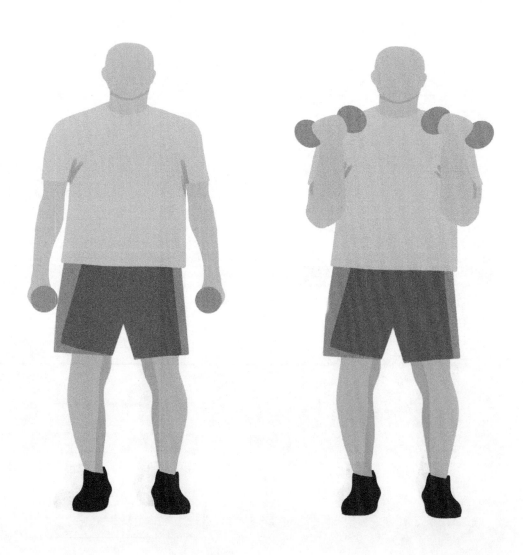

One-arm row (5-10 reps each side) (2-3 sets)

1. Find a secure surface where to stand on.

2. At approximately 45 degrees, bend at your waist while placing your hand on a secure surface. Remember to do this with feet shoulder-width apart.

3. Hold your weight with your free arm extended and almost perpendicular to the ground.

4. While doing these, slowly draw your elbow straight back, keeping the arm close to the body until your hand weight touches the body.

5. Hold the pose for a second. Then, you can slowly return to your starting position. Inhale as you return.

Do the other side.

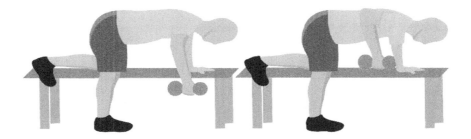

Seated Lateral Raise (5-10 reps) (2-3 sets)

1. Get a chair without the armrests.

2. Sit on it and ensure that the small of your back is pushed firmly against the chair's back.

3. Straighten your body, shoulders back. Plant your feet firmly on the ground, shoulder-width apart.

4. Using weights on each hand with arms at your side, please form a 90-degree angle between your upper arm and forearm. Note that this will be your starting position.

5. Inhale and exhale as you raise your elbows slowly out to your side. Hold the pose for one second.

6. Slowly, you can return to the starting position, inhaling as you return.

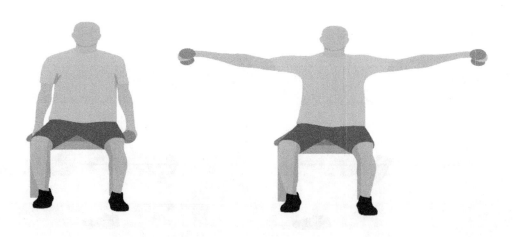

Tip: Your focus should be onward, with your chin up and away from your chest.

Glute Bridge Exercise (5-10 reps) (2-3 sets)

1. Lie on your back with your knees bent.

2. Tighten the muscles in your stomach.

3. Raise your hips off the floor until they line up with your knees and shoulders. Hold for three deep breaths.

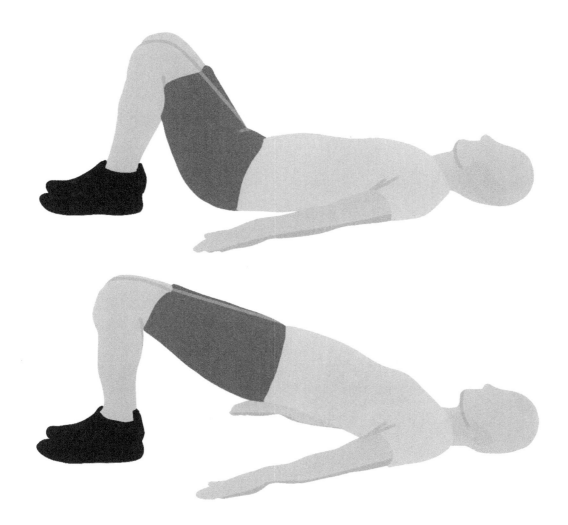

Bird Dog (5-10 reps each leg) (2-3 sets)

1. Start on your hands and knees with the hands under the shoulders and the knees under the hips.

2. Extend one leg and the opposite arm at the same time.

3. Pause for 3 to 5 seconds, return to the starting position, and switch sides.

4. Continue alternating sides until set is complete

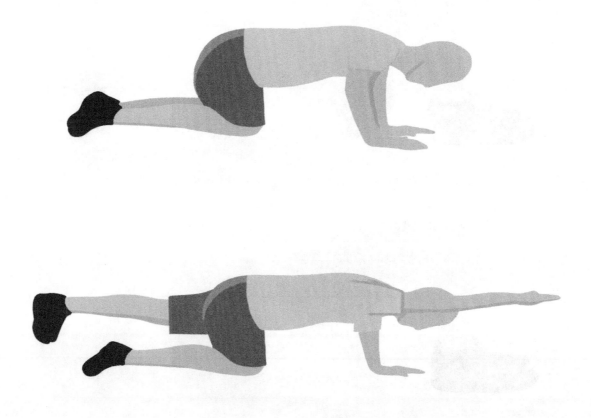

Kneeling Shoulder Tap Push Up (5-10 reps) (2-3 sets)

1. From your knees, place your hands on the ground, shoulder width apart.

2. Push your back up with the palms of your hands.

3. Repeat the push up but as you rise tap left hand on right shoulder. Keep abs tight throughout and avoid the torso "tipping" to the side as you tap.

4. Repeat, tapping the opposite shoulder.

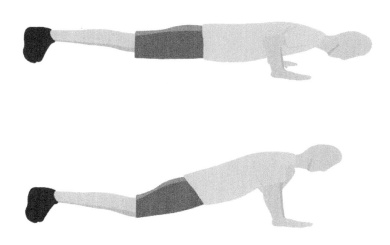

Mid Back Extension (5-10 reps) (2-3 sets)

1. Lie on a mat on your stomach and straighten your legs behind you. Place your elbows on the ground and slide your shoulders down.

2. Lift your upper back, pressing your hips into the mat. Keep your head and neck neutral. Hold for 30 seconds.

3. Lower to starting position. Complete 3 sets.

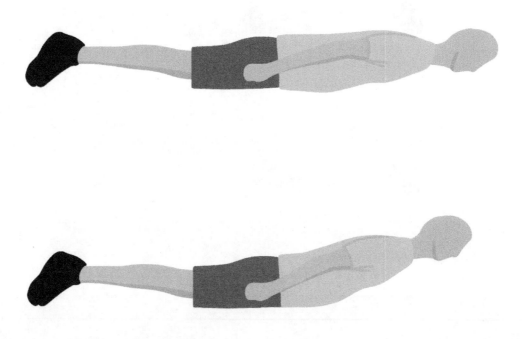

Sit Ups (7-10 reps) (2-3 sets)

1. Lie on your back on a mat with knees bent and feet flat on the floor.

2. Cross your arms in front of your chest.

3. Crunch your ab muscles to lift your shoulders off the mat.

4. Hold for a second, then slowly come back down to starting position.

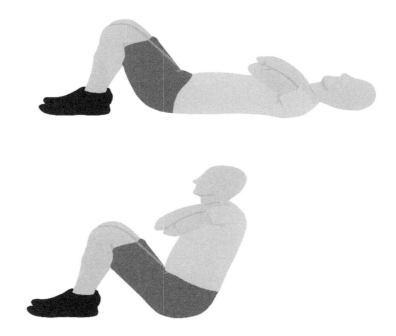

Lower Body Exercises

Squat Curl Knee Lift (5-10 reps each leg) (2-3 sets)

1. Start in squat position, weight back on heels and arms long next to side holding dumbbells.

2. Squeeze your glutes to press up and lift right knee as you curl the weights to your shoulders.

3. Slowly lower the weights back down and return to squat position. Repeat with left knee.

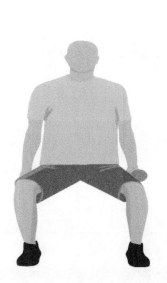
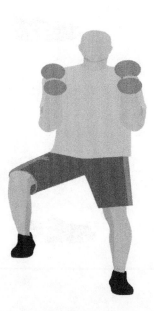

Calf Raises (5-10 reps) (2-3 sets)

1. Stand with your torso upright, your feet hip-width apart, and your toes pointing forward.

2. Raise your heels off the floor and squeeze your calves.

3. Return to the starting position, by slowly lowering your heels, and repeat.

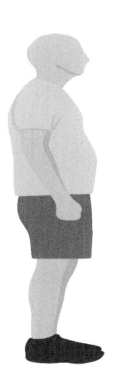 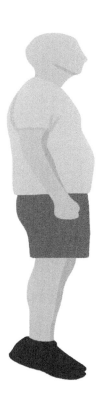

Half Squats (5-10 reps) (2-3 sets)

1. Bending your legs, push your butt back to a 45-degree angle, making sure not to position yourself in a full sit.

2. Extend your arms straight in front of you.

3. Pause for a second, then slowly raise your body back up by pushing through your heels.

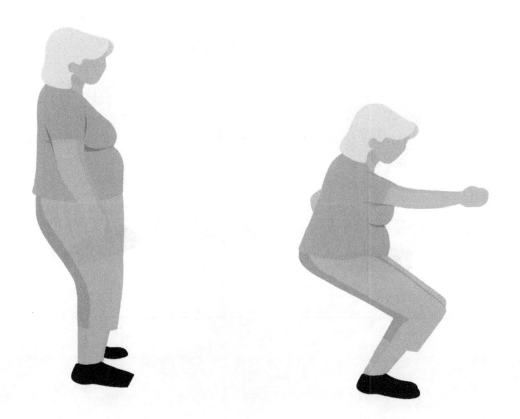

Step Up Exercise (7-10 reps each leg) (2-3 sets)

1. Pushing primarily through your lead foot, lift your body up onto the step.

2. Then step backward to the starting position.

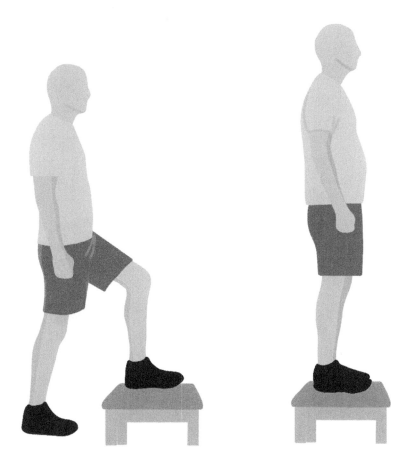

Tip: When you're doing step-ups, keep your back straight and your abdominal muscles nice and tight. Make sure your foot is planted entirely on the step

Squat Hold (5-10 reps) (2-3 sets)

1. Stand on your feet, hip-wide.

2. Bend knees lowering until the quads are parallel to the ground.

3. Stay in this position a few 5-10 seconds

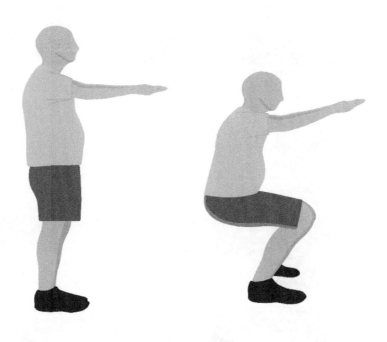

One of the main reasons for injury among seniors is falls. You don't have to succumb to slips and falls, though. Working out will strengthen your body and improve your balance, allowing you to walk more poise and confidently.

You can follow the above intermediate warm-ups, stretches, and exercises to ensure strength and flexibility in your later years.

Ready for a challenge? If your body permits, you can move on to more advanced workouts. Tune in for the next chapter!

Chapter 11
Advanced Workout

You can still partake in advanced workout routines even at an advanced age. They are a tad more difficult than the previous ones. But you can be assured of the best results.

Just a reminder, though. These workouts may not apply to people with some mobility and health issues. So, it's best to consult with your doctor to check if your body can meet the requirements.

The Warm Up

Arm Twists (10 reps)

1. Bring your arms out and away from your body until they form a straight, horizontal line parallel to the floor; keeping your palms facing down.

2. Rotate at the wrists and elbows leading up with your thumbs. Continue to rotate until your palms are facing up.

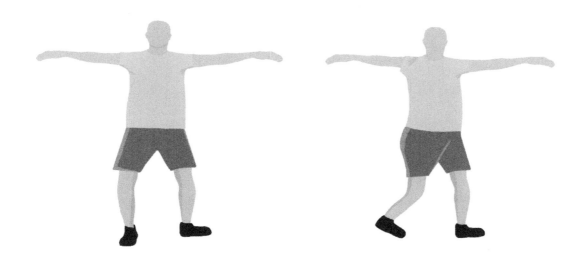

High stepping (30 seconds)

Run in place while pulling your knees as high as possible with each step. Keep your back straight do it as fast as you can breathe regularly you.

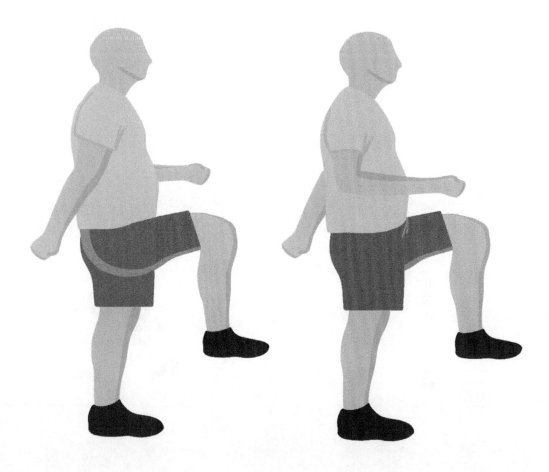

Heel to Toe Walk (20 steps)

1. Position the heel of one foot just in front of the toes of the other foot. Your heel and toes should touch or almost touch.

2. Choose a spot ahead of you and focus on it to keep you steady as you walk.

3. Take a step. Put your heel just in front of the toe of your other foot.

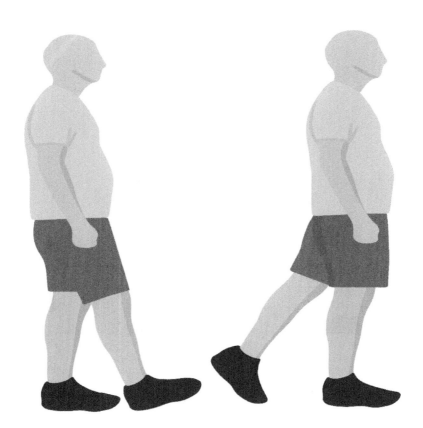

Tip: If you require assistance, go in a hallway or at the side of a counter.

Standing Hip Flexor (10 reps, each leg)

1. Stand with your legs shoulder width apart.

2. Hold onto a stable chair or table for support.

3. Keep your knee straight, toes pointed and kick your leg forward in a slow and controlled motion.

4. Return to the starting position.

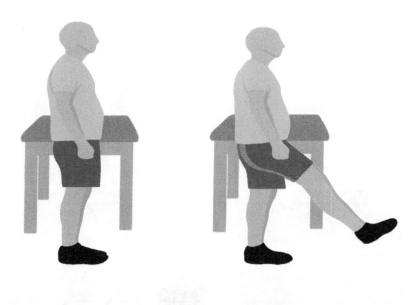

Tip: Perform an abdominal draw in to protect your back from injury. Do this by pulling your umbilicus (belly button) in towards your back.

Stretching

Calf Stretch (5-10 reps each leg)

1. Put your hands on a wall.

2. Stand in a lunge position.

3. Bend your front leg.

4. Shift your weight forward onto the front leg.

5. Press your back heel into the floor.

6. Repeat with the opposite leg in front.

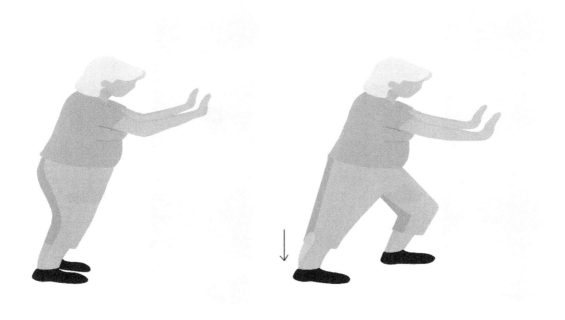

Reminder: Discontinue instantly if you feel pain in your Achilles tendon. That's where the calf attaches to the ankle.

Leg Swings (5-10 reps, each leg)

1. Start by standing on one leg, and swing the other leg forward and back. Use small swings that progress into larger swings as tolerated.

2. Then switch to side-to-side leg swings. This stretches the calf, quadriceps, hamstrings and groin muscle.

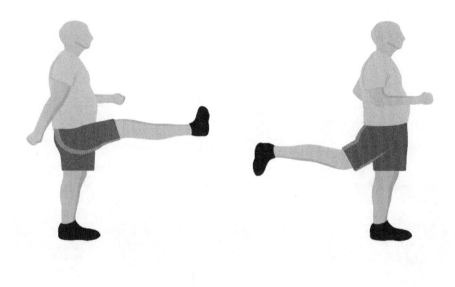

Tip: Begin with smaller swings and increase each size as your muscles become more flexible.

Seated Hamstring Stretch (5-10 reps, each leg)

1. Sit with one leg extended and your back straight. Bend your other leg.

2. Reach toward your ankle. Keep your knee, neck, and back straight.

3. Feel the stretch in the back of your thigh.

4. Hold for 30 to 60 seconds.

5. Repeat with the other leg.

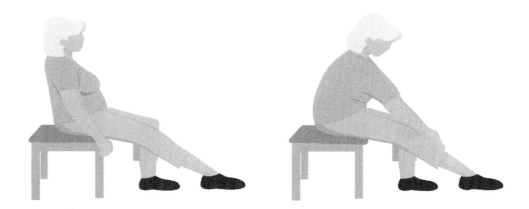

Glute Stretch (5-10 reps, each leg)

1. Lie flat on your back and bend both knees.

2. Gently pull the left leg toward you until you feel a stretch in your glutes.

3. Hold the stretch for 30 seconds and repeat with the other leg.

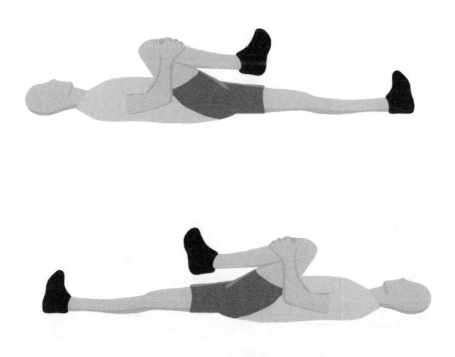

Tip: Stretch gently; overstretching might make your muscles stiffer.

Neck Circles (30 seconds)

1. Begin with your head straight and looking forward.

2. Gently tilt your head to the right and start rolling it back.

3. Keep rolling your head to the left and then down

4. Bring your head up to the starting position and repeat in the opposite direction.

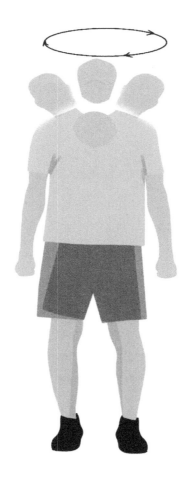

Tip: It's natural to feel tighter on one side than the other. On the side that feels tighter, try holding the stretch for a little longer.

Chest Stretch (5-7 reps)

1. Stand in an open doorway. Raise each arm up to the side, bent at 90-degree angles with palms forward.

2. Slowly step forward with one foot. Feel the stretch in your shoulders and chest.

3. Hold for 30 seconds. Step back and relax.

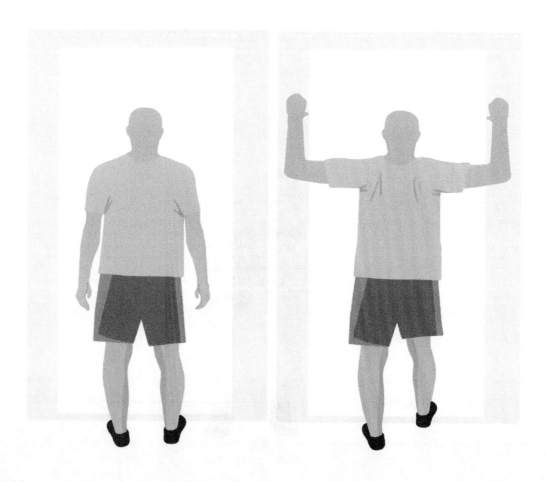

Standing Quadriceps Stretch (5 reps each leg)

1. Stand near a wall or a piece of sturdy exercise equipment for support.

2. Grasp your ankle and gently pull your heel up and back until you feel a stretch in the front of your thigh

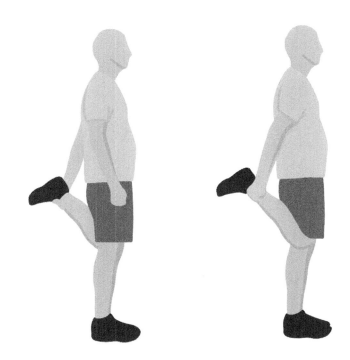

Upper Body Exercises

Push-ups (5 to 10 reps) (2-3 sets)

1. Get down on all fours, placing your hands slightly wider than your shoulders.

2. Straighten your arms and legs.

3. Lower your body until your chest nearly touches the floor.

4. Pause, then push yourself back up.

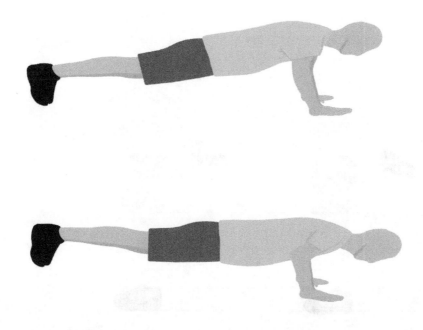

Row Exercise (10 reps) (2-3 sets)

1. Grab a set of dumbbells, bend your torso forward and keep your knees slightly bent.

2. Pull the dumbbells toward your waistline, while squeezing your shoulder blades.

3. Slowly lower the weights to the starting position.

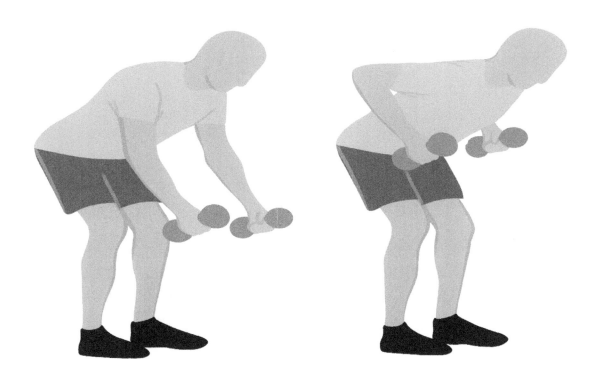

Shoulder Squeeze (10-12 reps) (2-3 sets)

1. Stand tall with feet hip-width apart. While pulling your elbows back and down.

2. Squeeze your shoulder blades together. Imagine you're squeezing a lemon between your shoulder blades.

3. Pause, then release. That's one rep.

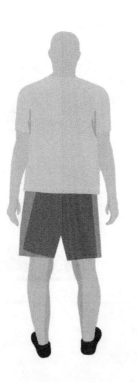 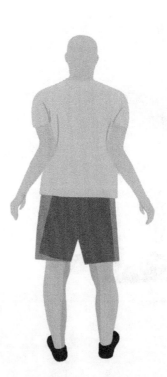

Hammer Curls (7-10 reps) (2-3 sets)

1. Grab a pair of dumbbells, and stand with your feet hip-width apart, arms at your sides, and palms facing in toward your body.

2. Keeping your torso stationary and elbows tucked close to your sides, bend your elbows (not your wrists) to curl the weights up to your shoulders.

3. Pause, then slowly return to start. That's one rep.

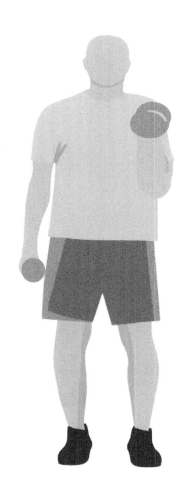
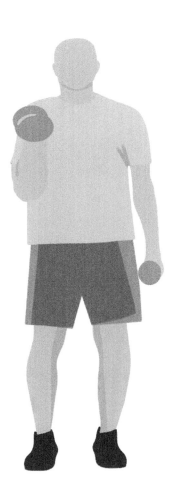

Triceps Extension (7-10 reps) (2-3 sets)

1. Stand with your feet hip-width apart, and hold the end of one dumbbell with both hands.

2. Position your arms so your elbows are pointing up, your upper arms are by your ears, and the dumbbell is behind your head. Your neck should be in line with your back, and your shoulders down and back.

3. Keeping your upper arms still, straighten your elbows so the dumbbell is above your head. Pause, and then slowly lower to return to start. That's one rep.

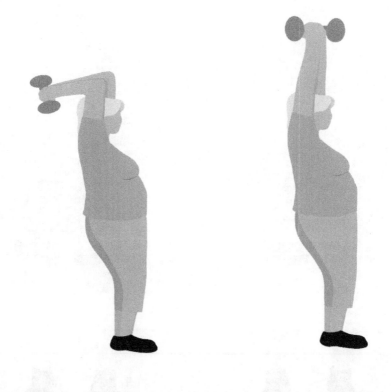

Diagonal Shoulder Raise with Resistance Band
(10-12 reps) (2-3 sets)

1. Take the resistance band underneath the opposite foot of the target limb.

2. The target limb is palm facing to the opposite hip.

3. Driving from the shoulder, pull the band across the body with a soft elbow.

4. The direction of the movement is a diagonal pull.

5. Slowly return to the start position.

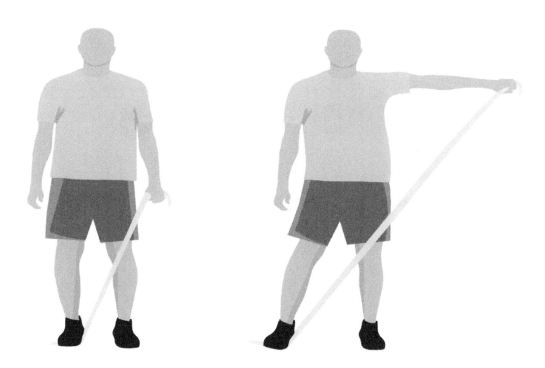

Triceps Kickback (10-12 reps) (2-3 sets)

(Do this Triceps exercise if unable to lift your hands above your head)

1. Start in a hip hinge position with your feet hip-width apart, knees slightly bent, and torso bent at a 45-degree angle.

2. Hold a dumbbell in each hand or simply make a fist. Bend your elbows so your upper arms are in line with your torso.

3. Keeping your upper arms steady, gently push your hands back to straighten your arms. Pause, then bend your arms back to return to start. That's one rep.

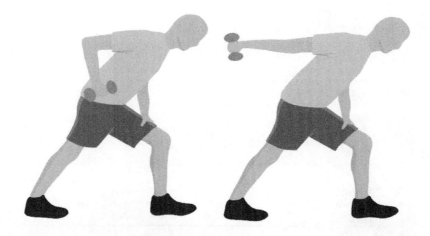

Upright Rows (10-12 reps) (2-3 sets)

1. Stand upright with your feet shoulder width apart.

2. Grasp a barbell with your palms facing downward and your hands closer than shoulder width apart.

3. Keep your arms extended downward with your elbows slightly bent so that the barbell is touching your upper legs. This is your starting position.

4. Keeping the barbell close to your body, exhale and raise the barbell straight up to your chest.

5. Hold for a moment and then reverse the motion back to the starting position.

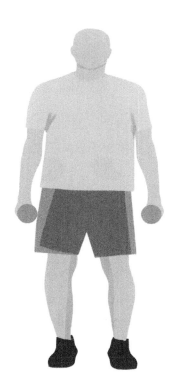
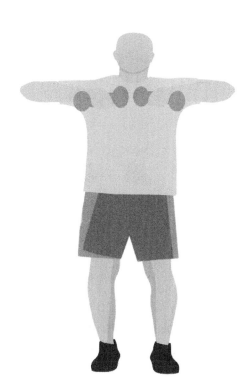

Shoulder Press (10-12 reps) (2-3 sets)

1. Exhale as you raise the weights above the head in a controlled motion.

2. Pause briefly at the top of the motion.

3. Inhale and return the dumbbells to the shoulders.

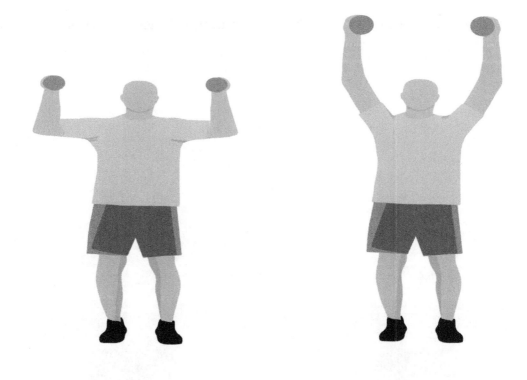

Tip: For your safety the lifting must be directly above the shoulders. Avoid letting the arms drift back, which could force the back to arch. Do this exercise while seated if you find it challenging to maintain excellent posture.

Lower Body Exercises

Goblet Squat (10-12 reps) (2-3 sets)

1. Hold the weight in front of your chest with both hands.

2. As you squat down, your elbows will track between your knees while the weight follows. (Alternate Exercise: Use a chair)

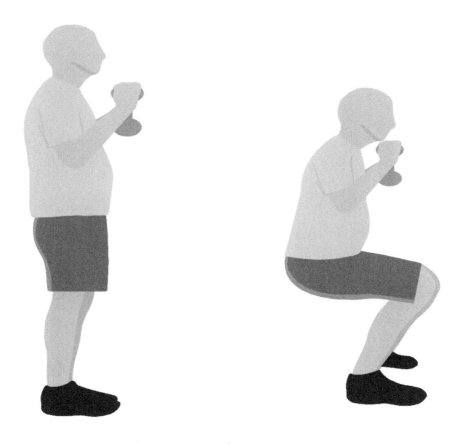

Tip: You may also do this by sitting down in a chair

Lunges

Walking lunges (10 reps for each leg) (2-3 sets)

1. With your weight evenly distributed, take a forward step with one leg. Your opposite knee should be bent until it almost touches the floor.

2. Straighten your knees and stand up again. Returning to an upright stance, take your first foot to meet your other foot.

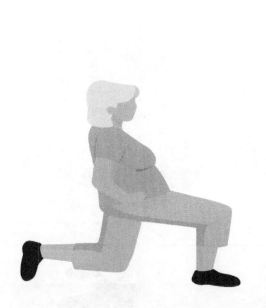
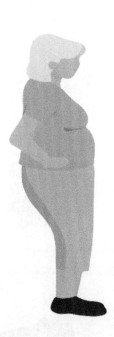

Straight leg raise (10-12 reps, each leg) (2-3 sets)

1. Lay down with your legs and back flat against floor.

2. Keep your arms on your sides.

3. Now keep your legs straight and raise your left leg with feet up until pointing straight in the air.

4. Slowly lower back down to the floor.

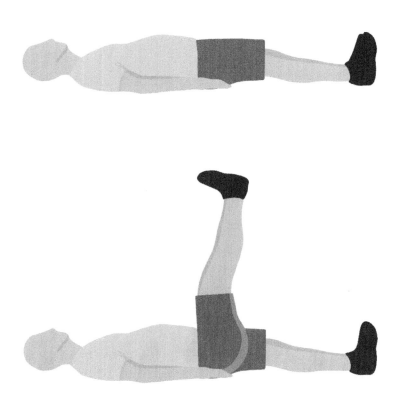

Toe Touch Jumping Jacks (2-3 sets)

1. Perform a modified jumping jack, without the jumping, by tapping your feet four to six inches out to the side one at a time.

2. Tap to the right 7 times and left 7 times for a total of 14 taps.

3. Pause, then repeat for 2 more rounds.

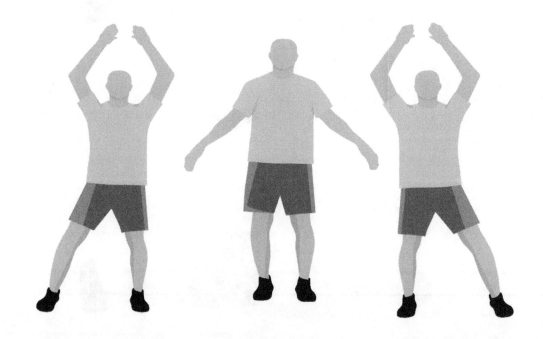

Side Squat (10 reps) (2-3 sets)

1. Stand tall with your feet together and hands on your hips.

2. Step your left foot out to the side. As you land, lower into a squat, bending at your knees and hips.

3. From there, squeeze your butt and press through both heels to stand back up, bringing your right foot in to meet your left foot as you do.

4. Immediately step your left foot out to the side as you squat once again.

5. Perform 5 squats leading with the left leg.

6. Pause, then reverse directions with 5 squats leading with the right leg.

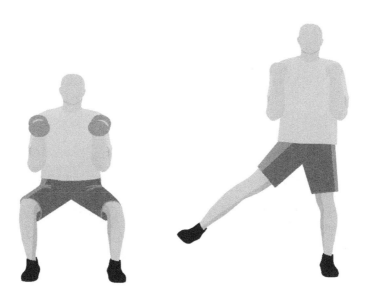

Tip:: When you squat into each repeat, maintain a straight back and an open chest. While you curl, keep the elbows tight to the ribcage.

Monster Walk (2-3 sets)

1. Place a resistance band around your legs, just above your knees.

2. Bend knees slightly with your feet hip-width apart.

3. Step to the right until the band provides resistance, then slide your left foot over to re-create your original stance.

4. Step to the right 7 times then to the left 7 times for a total of 14 reps.

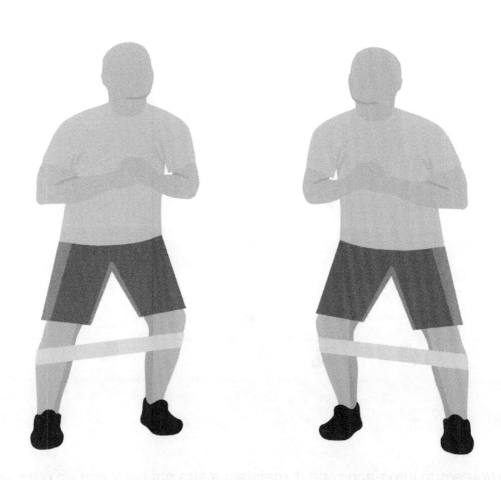

Floor Back Extension (8-10 reps) (2-3 sets)

1. Lie on the floor face-down. Extend your left arm straight overhead so that it aligns with your body. Keep the other arm at your side.

2. Slowly lift your left arm and right leg off the ground as you count to

3. Keep your arm and leg at the same level. Pause. Then slowly lower your arm and leg back to the ground.

4. Repeat 10 times for 1 set, and then switch to the right arm and the left leg for another 10 repetitions.

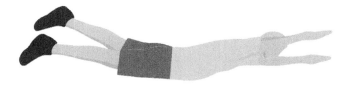

Forearm Plank

1. Lie face-down on the floor with your forearms on the ground. Your elbows should be directly under your shoulders and hands flat on the ground, elbow-width apart.

2. Engage your core to prepare. Then, press down through your forearms to raise your body off the floor until you're supported by your forearms and toes.

3. Keep your body in a straight line from your head down to your feet. Pull your navel into your spine and squeeze your glutes to keep your hips from dropping toward the floor.

4. Hold for 30 seconds or 1 minute if you're more advanced.

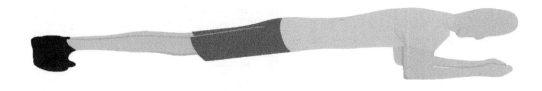

Modifications: Drop down to your knees if you can't keep your hips in line with your shoulders, or you feel pressure in your lower back.

Yes, these are more strenuous workouts. Yes, you are not getting any younger. But with the right amount of caution and if your body is capable, you can still do these activities.

Exercises for balance and strength are necessary, especially when you get older. It is simpler to perform daily tasks and less likely to stumble when you have strong muscles and better balance.

Apart from strength and balance, exercise helps improve cardiovascular health. Many activities are designed specifically for that purpose.

That's what we will delve into next.

Chapter 12
The Plateau

Anyone can encounter a workout plateau. Despite following up with your fitness routine, you may realize you're not losing weight, enhancing your strength, or building muscle. This may leave you feeling frustrated and unmotivated.

Fortunately, there are numerous strategies for overcoming a fitness plateau and advancing.

Breaking Through a Workout Plateau

A workout plateau happens when your body gets used to the rigors of your workouts. You can lose interest in working out, grow bored, or discover that you don't feel like it.

Repeating the same routines can diminish passion and motivation and result in a plateau. Overtraining, a lack of enough recuperation time, and burnout can all contribute to workout plateaus.

Other causes are:

    inefficient training methods

    not gradually working muscles

    uneven instruction

    unhealthy eating and living

    lack of sleep

If you experience it, don't worry. There are ways to overcome it.

1. Make little adjustments to your routine
You can induce a "training response" by changing the intensity, frequency, reps, utilization of different exercises, and many others. Making modest adjustments frequently allows your body to keep gaining strength while performing the same activities.

2. Measure your progress.

Keeping track of your fitness can help you determine if you've reached a plateau and what you can do to break it.

3. Hydrate

The effectiveness and recovery of muscles are greatly influenced by proper hydration. Even slight dehydration might result in headaches and decreased focus.

4. Prioritize nutrition

You may achieve your health and fitness goals through nutrition. You must consume adequate protein, carbs, healthy fats, and other micronutrients to gain muscle and recover rapidly. You may maximize the benefits of your workouts by establishing healthy eating habits.

5. Rest

Taking a break allows your body to recover and heal.

6. Utilize progressive overload

With this training method, your body is subjected to progressively more stress during workouts, forcing it to continue adapting.

7. Try something new

Give your body new challenges.

How to keep up

Here are some tips on how you can keep up with exercise:

Stay positive

Find activities that you enjoy.

Determine when and where best to exercise.

Make your workouts a habit.

Find a comfortable workout environment.

Avoid a sedentary lifestyle.

Look for ways to add more activity to your life.

How to improve

Here are some tips to ensure that you are advancing in your workouts toward better strength, flexibility, and balance:

1. Know that you will have setbacks. By preparing for them, you can make adjustments.
2. Consider pain.
As they say, "No pain; no gain."

3. Apply your workout to your body's capability.
A good exercise program targets your authentic self and not your ideal one.

4. Avoid exercise when hungry.
When hungry, you cannot perform at your best.

5. Don't shortchange your workouts.
Do the routines you least like first. That way, you are sure to finish because the ones you like are at the end.

6. Have variety in your workout.
A well-rounded program yields better results.

7. Motivate yourself.
Taking on a challenge is more manageable with a purpose or reward.

Don't be scared of a workout plateau. If it happens, you are ready for it.

Focus on improvement. Look forward to the results.

Now that you have all these exercise routines and health and fitness tips, you are ready to take on the challenge.

You may have misgivings as she did. But you can throw those out the window. It's time to choose the healthy route.

It's a new beginning.

It's time to begin an exercise program or make improvements to your current one.

It's not too late for Hayley.

For you.

For anyone.

What Can You Achieve with Your Energized Motivation?

There are so many exciting times ahead, from playing with the grandkids to taking that holiday you have been dreaming of.

Now, you know you have the confidence and physical abilities to enjoy life as a senior. Keep going on your strength training journey, because things will only get better. I have one small final ask, pass it on and help someone else to do the same!

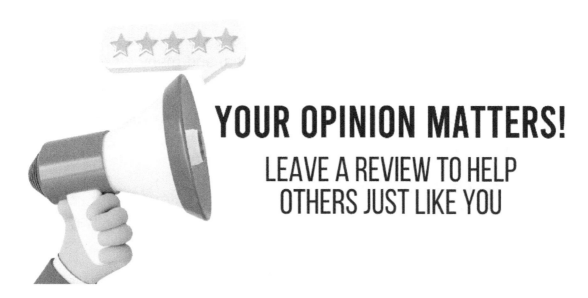

I promise it won't take more than a couple of minutes, but it could make years of difference to someone else. I will be forever grateful and I too would love to hear how you are progressing with your strength training and the amazing things you are accomplishing. Thank you and have fun!

Scan the QR code below to give your review

Conclusion

"Aging is just another word for living." - Cindy Joseph.

Aging is a part of life. Let's all accept that.

What you shouldn't accept is limiting yourself because of your age. Yes, your body is changing; your health is not what it used to be.

But in all this, you forget a crucial thing. There is a solution -

Exercise.

From improving strength to increasing confidence, exercise provides seniors with ample benefits. Cardiovascular diseases, diabetes, dementia, and many other health issues are aided through exercise.

It boosts our immunity and helps with weight management. Can you ask for more?

Do you want to be stronger? Do you want a better balance?

Choose an exercise that best fits your needs and go for it.

Include stretching, cardio, strength training, and other forms daily. Always adhere to a nutritious and balanced diet to double the chances of success.

Success in your health journey can be difficult if you don't have goals and things that motivate you. What are your health goals? What motivates you?

You now have different warm-up, stretching, and exercise ideas at your fingertips. All you need to do is take the first step.

Aim to engage in some form of physical activity each day, even if it is only for a short period. You'll be more inclined to follow your regimen if you do it this way.

Please remember that everyone has varying degrees of comfort with exercising. Starting slowly and creating a health plan specific to your capabilities is vital for your safety. Speaking of safety, always consult a health expert.

Most importantly, always remember that while making these constructive changes to your life, you must strive to enjoy yourself.

A crucial component of graceful aging is exercise. Regain your confidence by using the techniques you learned from this book.

Hayley claimed her life back. "Deciding to do home workouts is the best decision I have made in life," she said.

You should claim yours, too.

APPENDIX A
4-WEEK WORKOUT ROUTINES

Beginners with Limited Mobility
(Can be done for up to 4 weeks)

Workout A:

		Exercise	Sets	Reps	Rest B/W Sets
		Warmup			
1	Neck Turns	1	5 each turn	15 seconds
		Pre-Stretching			
2	Spine Twist	1	5 each side	15 seconds
3	Upper Back Stretch	1	5	15 seconds
		Exercises			
4	Seated Row (Resistance Bands)	2-3	5-10	1 minute
5	Bent over Row (Resistance Bands)	2-3	5-10	1 minute
6	Seated Arm Curls	2-3	10	1 minute
		Post-Stretching			
7	Seated Side Stretch	1	5	End of Workout

Workout B:

		Exercise	Sets	Reps	Rest B/W Sets
		Warmup			
1	Knee Lifts	1	10 each leg	15 seconds
		Pre-Stretching			
2	Seated Hip Stretch	1	5 each leg	15 seconds
3	Back of thigh Stretch or Knee to Chest	1	3-5 each side	15 seconds
		Exercises			
4	Extended Leg Raise	2-3	5-10	1 minute
5	Seated Hip Marching	2-3	5-10	1 minute
6	Toe Taps	2-3	10	1 minute
		Post-Stretching			
7	Ankle Rotations	1	3-5 each side	End of Workout

Workout C:

		Exercise	Sets	Reps	Rest B/W Sets
		Warmup			
1	Tummy Twists	1	10 each side	15 seconds
		Pre-Stretching			
2	Seated Backbend	1	5	15 seconds
3	Chest Stretch	1	3-5	15 seconds
		Exercises			
4	Chair Pushups	2-3	7-10	1 minute
5	Banded Chest Press (Resistance Bands)	2-3	5-10	1 minute
6	Bicep Curls (Resistance Bands)	2-3	10	1 minute
		Post-Stretching			
7	Seated Overhead Stretch	1	5	End of Workout

Beginners with Moderate Mobility
(Can be done for up to 4 weeks)

Workout A:

	Exercise	Sets	Reps	Rest B/W Sets
	Warmup			
1	Hip Circles	1	5-10	15 seconds
	Pre-Stretching			
2	Spine Twist	1	5 each side	15 seconds
3	Upper Back Stretch	1	5	15 seconds
	Exercises			
4	Modified Burpees	2-3	5-10	1 minute
5	Standing Hamstring Curl	2-3	5-10	1 minute
6	Chair Lunges	2-3	5-10 each leg	1 minute
7	Modified Chair Plank	2-3	10	1 minute
	Post-Stretching			
8	Seated Side Stretch	1	5	End of Workout

Workout B:

	Exercise	Sets	Reps	Rest B/W Sets
	Warmup			
1	Calf Raises	1	10	15 seconds
	Pre-Stretching			
2	Seated Hip Stretch	1	5 each leg	15 seconds
3	Back of thigh Stretch or Knee to Chest	1	3-5 each side	15 seconds
	Exercises			
4	Partial Squats	2-3	5-10	1 minute
5	Sit and Stand Squats	2-3	5-10	1 minute
6	Leg Extensions	2-3	5-10	1 minute
7	Seated Leg Extension (Resistance Bands)	2-3	10	1 minute
	Post-Stretching			
8	Ankle Rotations	1	3-5 each side	End of Workout

Workout C:

	Exercise	Sets	Reps	Rest B/W Sets
	Warmup			
1	Ankle Circles	1	5 for each foot	15 seconds
	Pre-Stretching			
2	Seated Backbend	1	5	15 seconds
3	Chest Stretch	1	3-5	15 seconds
	Exercises			
4	Wall Pushups	2-3	5-7	1 minute
5	Chest Pull (Resistance Bands)	2-3	5-10	1 minute
6	Band Triceps Pull (Resistance Bands)	2-3	10	1 minute
	Post-Stretching			
7	Seated Overhead Stretch	1	5	End of Workout

Intermediate Workout
(Can be done for up to 4 weeks)

Workout A:

	Exercise	Sets	Reps	Rest B/W Sets
		Warmup		
1	Hip Circles	1	5-10	15 seconds
		Pre-Stretching		
2	Chin Drop	1	5-7	15 seconds
		Exercises		
3	Bird Dog	2-3	5-10 each leg	1 minute
4	One-Arm Row	2-3	5-10 each side	1 minute
5	Glute Bridge	2-3	5-10	1 minute
6	Mid Back Extension	2-3	5-10	1 minute
7	Shoulder Shrugs	2-3	10-12	1 minute
		Post-Stretching		
8	Double-knee torso rotation	1	5	End of Workout

Workout B:

	Exercise	Sets	Reps	Rest B/W Sets
		Warmup		
1	Basic Squats	1	5-10	15 seconds
		Pre-Stretching		
2	Hula Hoop Hip Stretches	1	5-10 rotations	15 seconds
		Exercises		
3	Squat Curl Knee Lift	2-3	5-10 each leg	1 minute
4	Half Squats	2-3	5-10	1 minute
5	Squat Hold	2-3	5-10	1 minute
6	Calf Raises	2-3	5-10	1 minute
7	Step up	2-3	7-10 each leg	1 minute
		Post-Stretching		
8	Standing Squat Stretch	1	5-10	End of Workout

Workout C:

	Exercise	Sets	Reps	Rest B/W Sets
		Warmup		
1	Ankle Circles	1	5 for each foot	15 seconds
		Pre-Stretching		
2	Shoulder Stretch	1	5 each side	15 seconds
		Exercises		
3	Kneeling Shoulder Tap Pushup	2-3	5-10	1 minute
4	Shoulder Overhead Press	2-3	10-12	1 minute
5	Seated Lateral Raise	2-3	5-10	1 minute
6	Dumbbell Curl	2-3	10-12	1 minute
7	Situps	2-3	7-10	1 minute
		Post-Stretching		
8	Arm Opener	1	5-7	End of Workout

Advanced Workout
(Can be done for up to 4 weeks)

Workout A:

	Exercise	Sets	Reps	Rest B/W Sets
	Warmup			
1	Standing Hip Flexor	1	10 each leg	15 seconds
	Pre-Stretching			
2	Leg Swings	1	5-7	15 seconds
3	High Stepping	1	30 seconds	15 seconds
	Exercises			
4	Shoulder Squeeze	2-3	10-12	1 minute
5	Rows	2-3	10	1 minute
6	Upright Row	2-3	10-12	1 minute
7	Floor Back Extension	2-3	8-10	1 minute
8	Hammer Curls	2-3	10-12	1 minute
	Post-Stretching			
9	Glute Stretch	1	5	End of Workout

Workout B:

	Exercise	Sets	Reps	Rest B/W Sets
	Warmup			
1	Hipping Step	1	30 seconds	15 seconds
	Pre-Stretching			
2	Standing Quadriceps Stretch	1	5 each leg	15 seconds
3	Calf Stretch	1	5-10 each leg	15 seconds
	Exercises			
4	Goblet Squat	2-3	10-12	1 minute
5	Side Squat	2-3	10	1 minute
6	Toe Touch Jumping Jacks OR Monster Walks	2-3	14	1 minute
7	Walking Lunges	2-3	10 each leg	1 minute
8	Straight Leg Raise	2-3	10-12 each leg	1 minute
	Post-Stretching			
9	Seated Hamstring Stretch	1	5-10	End of Workout

Workout C:

	Exercise	Sets	Reps	Rest B/W Sets
		Warmup		
1	Arm Circles	1	10	15 seconds
		Pre-Stretching		
2	Chest Stretch	1	5-7	15 seconds
		Exercises		
3	Push-ups	2-3	5-10	1 minute
4	Shoulder Press	2-3	10-12	1 minute
5	Diagonal Shoulder Raise (Resistance Band)	2-3	10-12	1 minute
6	Tricep Kickback	2-3	10-12	1 minute
7	Tricep Extension	2-3	7-10	1 minute
8	Forearm Plank	1	30-60 seconds	1 minute
		Post-Stretching		
9	Neck Circles	1	5-7	End of Workout

References:

5 ways to Stop dwelling on Negative thoughts. (n.d.). happify.com. https://www.happify.com/hd/stop-dwelling-on-negative-thoughts/

12 Best Shoulder Exercises For Seniors And The Elderly. (n.d.). ELDERGYM®. https://eldergym.com/shoulder-exercises/

Batsis, J. A., & Zagaria, A. B. (2018). Addressing obesity in aging patients. Medical Clinics of North America, 102(1), 65–85. https://doi.org/10.1016/j.mcna.2017.08.007

Bsn, M. D. R. (2018, September 29). Everything you should know about oxidative stress. Healthline. https://www.healthline.com/health/oxidative-stress

Cancer Research UK. (2021, August 11). Age and cancer. https://www.cancerresearchuk.org/about-cancer/causes-of-cancer/age-and-cancer#:~:text=But%20as%20we%20get%20older,can%20sometimes%20lead%20to%20cancer.

Collagen vs elastin: Know the difference. (2021, November 10). SkinKraft. https://skinkraft.com/blogs/articles/collagen-vs-elastin

Cpt, P. W. (2022). Why Aren't You Motivated to Exercise? Verywell Fit. https://www.verywellfit.com/why-arent-you-motivated-to-exercise-1231389#toc-no-motivation-to-workout

Cpt, P. W. (2022b). Why Aren't You Motivated to Exercise? Verywell Fit. https://www.verywellfit.com/why-arent-you-motivated-to-exercise-1231389#toc-no-motivation-to-workout

Cronkleton, E. (2022, April 29). Hit a workout plateau? Here's how to get through it. Healthline. https://www.healthline.com/nutrition/workout-plateau#why-it-happens

DailyCaring. (2023). 10 reasons why seniors lose their appetite. DailyCaring. https://dailycaring.com/why-do-seniors-lose-their-appetites/

Diaphragm and lungs: MedlinePlus Medical Encyclopedia Image. (n.d.). https://medlineplus.gov/ency/imagepages/19380.htm#:~:text=The%20diaphragm%2C%20located%20below%20the,and%20the%20chest%20cavity%20enlarges.

Duncan, A. (n.d.). Don't skip the warm-up: injury prevention and workout performance. https://www.nifs.org/blog/the-importance-of-a-warm-up-for-injury-prevention-and-workout-performance

Estrogen's effects on the female body. (2022, November 1). Johns Hopkins Medicine. https://www.hopkinsmedicine.org/health/conditions-and-diseases/estrogens-effects-on-the-female-body#:~:text=What%20is%20estrogen%3F,small%20amounts%20of%20the%20hormones.

Falls and Fractures in Older Adults: Causes and Prevention. (n.d.). National Institute on Aging. https://www.nia.nih.gov/health/falls-and-fractures-older-adults-causes-and-prevention#:~:text=Age%2Drelated%20loss%20of%20muscle,all%20risk%20factors%20for%20falling.

Flexibility exercise (Stretching). (2023, January 24). www.heart.org. https://www.heart.org/en/healthy-living/fitness/fitness-basics/flexibility-exercise-stretching

Graber, E. (2020). Which to choose: full-fat, low-fat, or non-fat dairy? American Society for Nutrition. https://nutrition.org/which-to-choose-full-fat-low-fat-or-non-fat-dairy/

Harvard Brain Initiative. (2021, April 14). How aging affects blood flow to the brain - Harvard Brain Science Initiative. Harvard Brain Science Initiative. https://brain.harvard.edu/hbi_news/how-aging-affects-blood-flow-to-the-brain/

Harvard Health. (2021, March 6). Foods linked to better brainpower. https://www.health.harvard.edu/healthbeat/foods-linked-to-better-brainpower

How much should I eat? Quantity and quality. (n.d.). National Institute on Aging. https://www.nia.nih.gov/health/how-much-should-i-eat-quantity-and-quality#portion

Inhc, A. C. A. (2021). How to do the Overhead Side Reach Stretch. Verywell Fit. https://www.verywellfit.com/how-to-do-the-overhead-side-reach-stretch-5090400#:~:text=The%20overhead%20side%20reach%20stretch%20in%20particular%20stretches%20your%20back,gentle%20pressure%20that%20eases%20soreness.

Killoran, E. (2022). How To Read Food Labels – 10 Tips. Pritikin Health Resort. https://www.pritikin.com/your-health/healthy-living/eating-right/food-labels.html

Lactose intolerance - Symptoms & causes - Mayo Clinic. (2022, March 5). Mayo Clinic. https://www.mayoclinic.org/diseases-conditions/lactose-intolerance/symptoms-causes/syc-20374232

Mayo Clinic Staff. (2022, February 12). Stretching: Focus on flexibility. Mayo Cinic. Retrieved July 21, 2023, from https://www.mayoclinic.org/healthy-lifestyle/fitness/in-depth/stretching/art-20047931

Patel, K. (2022, September 28). Vitamin E. Examine. Retrieved July 21, 2023, from https://examine.com/supplements/vitamin-e/

Physical activity. (2016, April 12). Obesity Prevention Source. https://www.hsph.harvard.edu/obesity-prevention-source/obesity-causes/physical-activity-and-obesity/

Physical activity. (2016b, April 12). Obesity Prevention Source. https://www.hsph.harvard.edu/obesity-prevention-source/obesity-causes/physical-activity-and-obesity/

Professional, C. C. M. (n.d.). Aerobic exercise. Cleveland Clinic. https://my.clevelandclinic.org/health/articles/7050-aerobic-exercise

Rd, A. W. P. (2019). What is Calcium? Food Insight. https://foodinsight.org/what-is-calcium/

Rd, K. J. M. (2019, April 26). 9 Health benefits of eating whole grains. Healthline. https://www.healthline.com/nutrition/9-benefits-of-whole-grains#TOC_TITLE_HDR_3

Rd, L. W. (2018, November 14). Boost your brain power with the right nutrition. The Ohio State University Wexner Medical Center. https://wexnermedical.osu.edu/blog/boost-your-brain-power-with-the-right-nutrition#:~:text=Fat%20is%20very%20important%20for,important%20for%20learning%20and%20memory.

Rockwell, R. (2020). The benefits of leg raise exercises. LIVESTRONG.COM. https://www.livestrong.com/article/525754-the-benefits-of-leg-raise-exercises/

Starting a Workout Routine. (2022, September 29). Cleveland Clinic. Retrieved July 21, 2023, from https://health.clevelandclinic.org/living-with-a-chronic-disease-4-best-tips-for-exercising/#:~:text=Choose%20low%2Dimpact%20aerobic%20activities,up%20without%20hurting%20your%20body.

Selenium. (2023, March 7). The Nutrition Source. https://www.hsph.harvard.edu/nutritionsource/selenium/#:~:text=Selenium%20is%20a%20component%20of,inflammation%20and%20other%20health%20problems.

Slide show: Add antioxidants to your diet. (2022, March 1). Mayo Clinic. https://www.

mayoclinic.org/healthy-lifestyle/nutrition-and-healthy-eating/multimedia/antioxidants/sls-20076428#:~:text=Antioxidants%20are%20substances%20that%20may,to%20tobacco%20smoke%20or%20radiation.

Strength training: Get stronger, leaner, healthier. (2023, April 29). Mayo Clinic. https://www.mayoclinic.org/healthy-lifestyle/fitness/in-depth/strength-training/art-20046670

Stretching: Focus on flexibility. (2022, February 12). Mayo Clinic. https://www.mayoclinic.org/healthy-lifestyle/fitness/in-depth/stretching/art-20047931

Vitamin B6: MedlinePlus Medical Encyclopedia. (n.d.). https://medlineplus.gov/ency/article/002402.htm

Vitamin D. (2023, March 7). The Nutrition Source. https://www.hsph.harvard.edu/nutritionsource/vitamin-d/#:~:text=It%20is%20a%20fat%2Dsoluble,control%20infections%20and%20reduce%20inflammation.

Watson, S. (2014, July 20). Balance training. WebMD. https://www.webmd.com/fitness-exercise/a-z/balance-training

What is Diabetes? (2023, April 24). Centers for Disease Control and Prevention. https://www.cdc.gov/diabetes/basics/diabetes.html#:~:text=With%20diabetes%2C%20your%20body%20doesn,vision%20loss%2C%20and%20kidney%20disease.

WebMD Editorial Contributors. (2021, March 24). What to know about dehydration in older adults. WebMD. https://www.webmd.com/healthy-aging/what-to-know-about-dehydration-in-older-adults

Wrinkles - Symptoms and causes - Mayo Clinic. (2023, January 21). Mayo Clinic. https://www.mayoclinic.org/diseases-conditions/wrinkles/symptoms-causes/syc-20354927

https://healthandhumansciences.fsu.edu/wp-content/uploads/2020/09/Health-Care-for-Older-Adults.pdf

Agrawals Fashion, Home & Decor, Vehicles. (2021, December 17). Strength training quote. Pinterest. https://www.pinterest.com/pin/strength-training-quote--954903927212516887/

Made in the USA
Las Vegas, NV
13 October 2024